The Recipes Book for Family

The Complete Cookbook to Lose Weight the Healthy Way

Odell Clayton

Table of Contents

Breakfast

Definitive Egg Salad

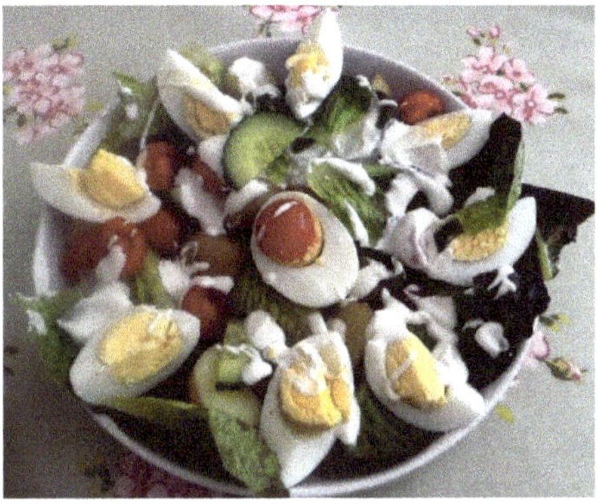

(Prepping time: 10 minutes | Cooking time: 5 minutes | For 4 servings)

Ingredients

- ¼ teaspoon pepper
- ½ teaspoon salt
- 1-piece dill
- 2 tablespoons mayonnaise
- ½ teaspoon Dijon mustard
- 2 tablespoons chives
- 4 whole eggs
- 2 hardboiled eggs

How To

1. Take a pan and fill it with water, add eggs, and place on high heat

2. Bring to a boil
3. Once eggs are done, drain water and add eggs to ice water bath
4. Once cooled, remove shells
5. Gently remove yolks from two eggs and slice them up
6. Add pepper, salt, mustard, dill, chives, and mayo to a bowl and stir well; add sliced up egg whites and egg yolks
7. Mix well
8. Enjoy!

Nutritional Values (Per Serving)

- Calories: 270
- Fat: 4g
- Carbohydrates: 55g
- Protein: 11g
- Saturated Fat: 1g
- Sodium: 129mg
- Fiber: 3g

Tri-Ingredient Pancake

(Prepping time: 10 minutes | Cooking time: 10 minutes | For 4 servings)

Ingredients

- 1 small-sized, ripe banana
- 1 medium-sized egg
- 2 tablespoons wholemeal, self-rising flour
- Cooking spray

How To

1. Take a medium-sized bowl and add banana, mashing it using the back of a spoon or a fork.
2. Whisk in egg and flour and mix well to combine everything.
3. Allow the mix to sit for 5 minutes.
4. Take a nonstick frying pan and grease it with oil. Heat the pan over medium heat and spoon in 2 tablespoons of batter for each pancake.
5. Cook for 2 minutes (each side) until the whole batter has been used up.
6. Keep repeating until all of the batters have been used up.
7. Enjoy!

Nutritional Values (Per Serving)

- Calories: 139
- Fat: 6g
- Carbohydrates: 18g
- Protein: 3g
- Saturated Fat: 2g
- Sodium: 221 mg
- Fiber: 2g

Banana Strawberry Overnight Oats

(Prepping Time: 10 mins | Cooking Time: 10 mins | For 2 servings)

Ingredients

- 1 banana, sliced
- 1 cup frozen strawberries
- 2 teaspoons honey
- ½ cup yogurt (dairy free)
- 2/3 cup silk almond milk
- 2/3 cup oats, rolled

How To

1. Heat strawberries in a saucepan to defrost them.
2. Mash them until they transform into a thick sauce.
3. Take out and let the mixture cool for a while.
4. Now, add honey, dairy-free yogurt, oats and silk almond milk in a bowl.
5. Then add strawberry sauce and mix well.
6. Seal the mixture in a container and place it in the refrigerator for a night.
7. Take out the strawberry oats and top them with sliced banana.
8. Serve and enjoy!

Nutritional Values (Per Serving)

- Calories: 266
- Fat: 3.6g
- Saturated Fat: 1g
- Trans Fat: 2.6g
- Carbohydrates: 51.2g
- Fiber: 6.1g
- Sodium: 99mg
- Protein: 8.1g

Granola and Yogurt Bowl

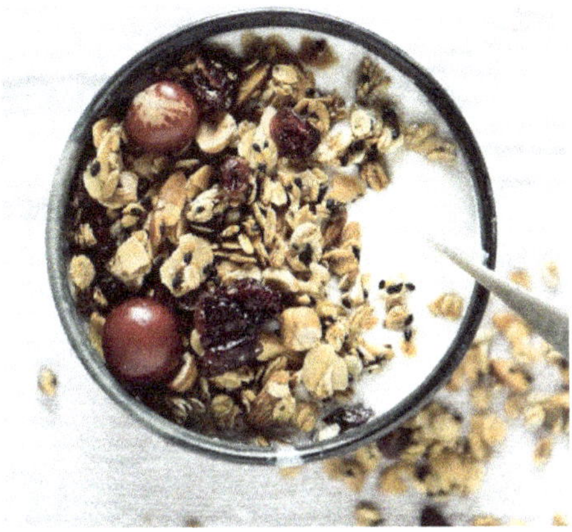

(Prepping Time: 5 min | Cooking Time: 0 min | For 2 servings)

Ingredients

- 2 tablespoons crunchy maple granola
- 2 tablespoons fresh raspberries
- 2 tablespoons fresh blueberries
- ¼ cup fresh strawberries, hulled and sliced
- 1 cup plain Greek yogurt (fat-free), divided

How To

1. Add all the berries in a bowl and mix well.
2. Pour half of the yogurt over the mixture and mix.
3. Now, pour the mixture in 2 glasses and place remaining yogurt over the berries.
4. Top with granola and serve.

Nutritional Values (Per Serving)

- Calories: 235
- Fat: 7.1g
- Saturated Fat: 0.5g
- Trans Fat: 5.1g
- Carbohydrates: 26.5g
- Fiber: 3.5g
- Sodium: 160mg
- Protein: 9.3g

Breakfast smoothie bowl

(Prepping Time: 15 minutes | Cooking Time: 20 minutes | For 6 servings)

Ingredients

- 6oz Keto Granola (Low Carb-No Sugar)
- 2 cups Low Fat Almond Non-Dairy Yogurt
- 1 teaspoon poppy seeds
- 1 teaspoon chia seeds
- 1 teaspoon flax seeds
- 3 ripe bananas, mashed
- 1 cup strawberries, washed, stemmed, and quartered
- 3 teaspoons cinnamon
- 3/4 teaspoon nutmeg
- 3 tablespoons sugar-free strawberry jam
- Pinch of salt

How To

1. Mix all of the ingredients apart from the strawberries, flax, chia, and poppy seeds, in a bowl.
2. Divide between 6 bowls
3. Top with strawberries, flax, chia, and poppy seeds, creating a nice pattern with the seeds on top of each bowl.
4. Serve immediately

Nutritional Values (Per Serving)

- Calories: 277
- Fat: 18.6g
- Saturated Fat: 7.1g
- Trans Fat: 0g
- Carbohydrates: 21.9g
- Fiber: 9g
- Sodium: 47mg
- Protein: 5.6g

Caramel Frappuccino

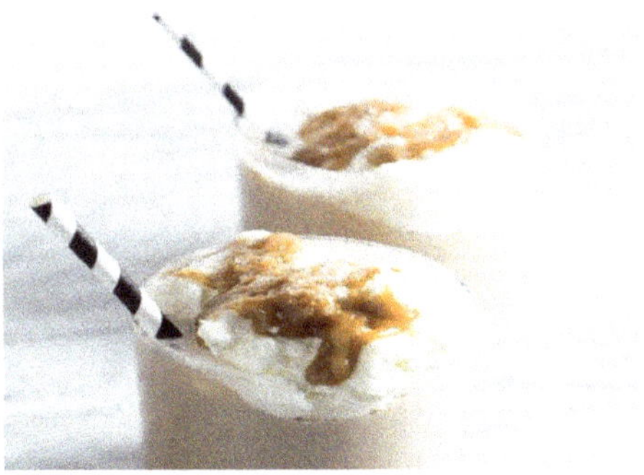

(Prepping Time: 1 minutes | Cooking Time: 1 min. | For 1 servings)

Ingredients

- 1/2 cup(s) soy milk
- 1/2 cup(s) prepared coffee, at room temperature
- 1 packet of Powdered Stevia
- 1 scoop protein powder
- 1 teaspoon(s) sugar free caramel syrup
- 6 ice cubes

How To

1. Put all the ingredients in a blender and pulse.
2. Serve in a tall chilled glass and enjoy!

Nutritional Values (Per Serving)

- Calories: 150
- Fat: 2.1g
- Saturated Fat: 0.3g
- Trans Fat: 0g
- Carbohydrates: 13.1g
- Fiber: 2.7g
- Sodium: 131mg
- Protein: 19.7g

Tropical Smoothie

(Prepping Time: 5 minutes | Cooking Time: 1 minute | For 8 servings)

Ingredients

- 1 cup(s) pineapple, in chunks
- 1 cup(s) mango, in chunks
- 1 banana
- 2 cup(s)s low fat milk
- 1 cup(s) low fat vanilla yogurt
- 2 scoops Protein Powder
- 8 ice cubes

How To

1. Place all of your ingredients in a blender and pulse until smooth
2. Serve cold

Nutritional Values (Per Serving)

- Calories: 117
- Fat: 2.5g
- Saturated Fat: 1.1g
- Trans Fat: 0.1g
- Carbohydrates: 18g
- Fiber: 1g
- Sodium: 65mg
- Protein: 7g

Hearty Onion Soup

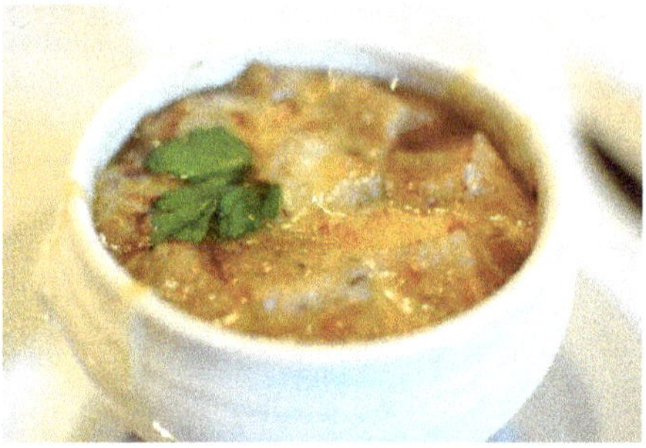

(Prepping time: 10 minutes | Cooking time: 25 minutes | For 4 servings)

Ingredients

- 2 large onions, finely sliced
- 2 cups vegetable stock
- 1 teaspoon brown sugar
- 1 cup red wine
- 1 measure brandy
- 1 teaspoon herbs de Provence
- 4 slices stale bread
- 4 ounces strong cheese, grated
- 1-ounce parmesan, grated
- 1 tablespoon plain flour
- 2 tablespoons olive oil
- 1-ounce butter
- Salt as needed
- Pepper as needed

How To

1. Take a pan and place it over medium-high heat.
2. Add oil and butter and allow it to heat up.

3. Add onion and sugar and keep cooking until the sugar dissolves and the onions are slightly caramelized.
4. Pour in brandy and flambé. Stir well to put out flames.
5. Add flour and herbs de Provence and stir.
6. Add stock, followed by the gradual addition of red Wine.
7. Season a bit and drop the heat to low.
8. Simmer for 20 minutes, adding a bit more water if needed to make it less thick.
9. Ladle the soup into bowls.
10. Place rounds of stale bread on top and add a bit of cheese.
11. Garnish with some parmesan.
12. Broil for just a bit to melt the cheese, then serve!

Nutritional Values (Per Serving)

- Calories: 55
- Fat: 1.7g
- Carbohydrates: 8g
- Protein: 3.6g
- Saturated Fat: 0.5g
- Sodium: 190 mg
- Fiber: 1g

The Berry Almond Chiller

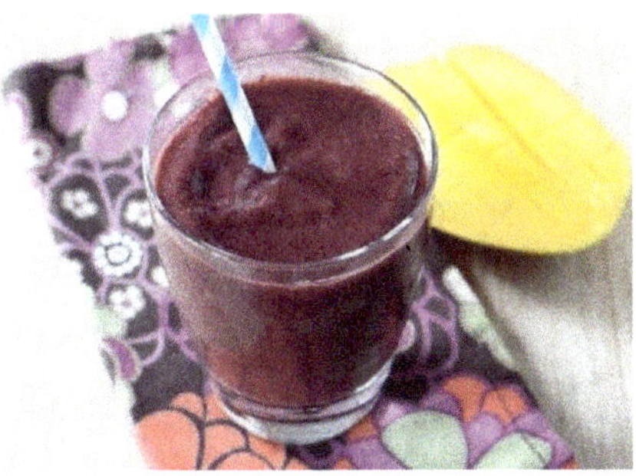

(Prepping time: 10 minutes | Cooking time: 0 minutes | For 4 servings)

Ingredients

- 1 cup frozen blueberries
- 1 whole banana
- ½ cup almond milk
- 1 tablespoon almond butter
- Water as needed

How To

1. Add the listed ingredients to your blender and blend them
2. Once you have a smooth mixture, chill and serve!

Nutritional Values (Per Serving)

- Calories: 321
- Fat: 11 g
- Saturated Fat: 4 g
- Carbohydrates: 55 g
- Fiber: 5 g
- Sodium: 78 mg
- Protein: 5 g

Blueberry Lemon Donuts

(Prepping Time: 15 minutes | Cooking Time: 10 minutes | For 10 Servings)

Ingredients

- 1 cup whole wheat flour
- 1/3 cup Splenda

- 3/4 teaspoon baking powder
- 3/4 teaspoon baking soda
- 1/4 teaspoon salt
- 1 egg
- 1/2 cup low-fat yogurt
- 1 tablespoon canola oil
- zest of one lemon
- 1 tablespoon lemon juice
- 1 1/2 cup fresh blueberries

How To

1. Preheat oven to 375F.
2. Spray a doughnut pan with cooking spray.
3. Mix all the dry ingredients in a bowl.
4. In a separate bowl, beat all the wet ingredients apart from the fruit.
5. Mix the dry mix with the wet until you get a smooth batter
6. Gently fold in the fruit
7. Drop 2 tablespoons in each donut mold
8. Bake for 10 minutes, until donuts are golden brown.

Nutritional Values (Per Serving):

- Calories: 118
- Fat: 2.2g
- Saturated Fat: 0.4g
- Trans Fat: 0.1g
- Carbohydrates: 20.2g
- Fiber: 0.9g
- Sodium: 170 mg
- Protein: 2.7g

Cinnamon Tea

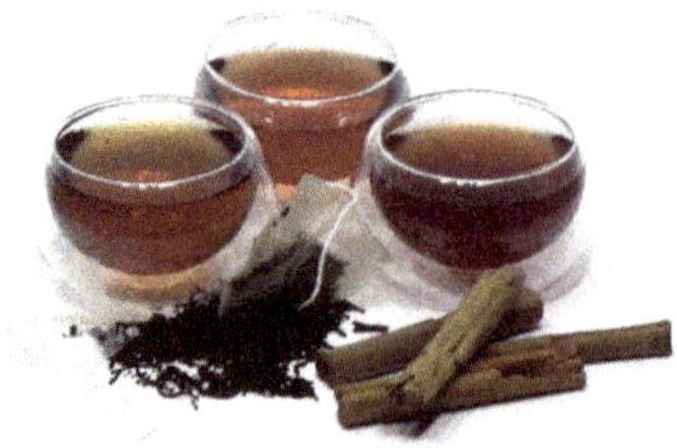

(Prepping Time: 10 min | Cooking Time: 5 min | For 2 Servings)

Ingredients

- 1 cup water
- 4 whole black peppercorns
- 1 teaspoon black tea
- ½ cup fat-free cream
- 2 cinnamon sticks

How To

1. Add water, peppercorns, and cinnamon in a saucepan. Boil well.
2. Now, reduce heat and let it simmer for some time.
3. Add cream, cook until smooth and strain the tea into 2 cups.
4. Serve hot and enjoy!

Nutritional Values (Per Serving)

- Calories: 25
- Fat: 0g

- Saturated Fat: 0g
- Trans Fat: 0g
- Carbohydrates: 5.9g
- Fiber: 1.3g

Grilled Peaches

(Prepping Time: 10 minutes | Cooking Time: 6 minutes | For 8 Servings)

Ingredients

- 4 peaches, halved
- 4 tablespoon honey
- 3 teaspoon cinnamon
- 1/2 teaspoon salt
- ½ tablespoon canola oil

How To

1. Preheat your oven grill.
2. In a bowl, mix the cinnamon, honey, salt, and oil
3. Dip peaches in the mixture
4. Arrange peaches cut side up on a baking dish lined with parchment paper and grill for 6 8 minutes.
5. Serve immediately

Nutritional Values (Per Serving)

- Calories: 71
- Fat: 1.1g
- Saturated Fat: 0.1g
- Trans Fat: 0g

- Carbohydrates: 16.3g
- Fiber: 1.6g
- Sodium: 146mg
- Protein: 0.8g

Chai Latte

Prepping Time: 5 minutes | Cooking Time: 5 minutes | For 8 Servings)

Ingredients

- 8 black tea bags
- 4 teaspoon(s) cinnamon
- 2 teaspoon(s) ginger, ground
- 1 teaspoon(s) allspice
- 4 cup(s)s of water
- 4 cup(s)s low fat milk
- 4 tablespoon(s) Powdered Stevia (or another sweetener)

How To

1. In a saucepan over high heat, add the water, the spices and the teabags.
2. Bring to a boil then strain.
3. Divide among the mugs.
4. In a separate saucepan add the milk and the sweetener. Cook until your sweetener has dissolved, about 4 minutes.
5. Divide among the mugs.
6. Serve hot topped with cinnamon.

Nutritional Values (Per Serving)

- Calories: 49
- Fat: 0.2g
- Saturated Fat: 0.1g
- Trans Fat: 0g
- Carbohydrates: 10g
- Fiber: 1g
- Sodium: 61mg
- Protein: 4g

Antioxidant Bomb Smoothie

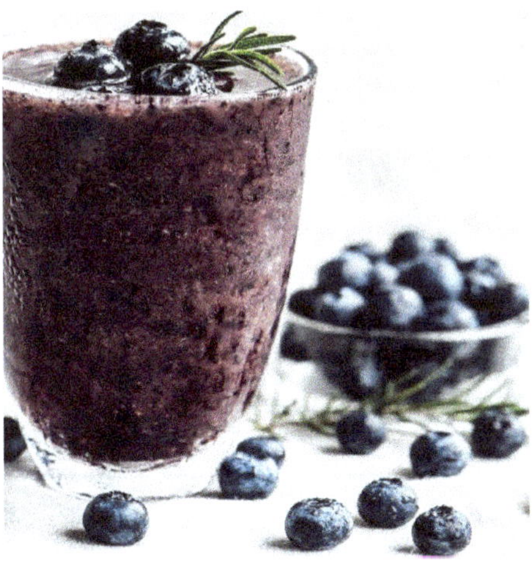

(Prepping Time: 5 minutes | Cooking Time: 1 minute | For 8 Servings)

Ingredients

- 1 cup(s) strawberries
- 1/2 cup(s) blueberries
- 1/2 cup(s) raspberries

- 1/2 cup(s) black currants
- 1/2 cup(s) red currants
- 2 cup(s)s low fat milk
- 1 cup(s) fat free vanilla yogurt
- 2 scoops Protein Powder
- 8 ice cubes

How To

1. Place all of your ingredients in a blender and pulse until smooth
2. Serve cold

Nutritional Values (Per Serving)

- Calories: 105
- Fat: 2.5g
- Saturated Fat: 1.1g
- Trans Fat: 0.1g
- Carbohydrates: 14g
- Fiber: 2g
- Sodium: 65mg
- Protein: 7g

Minty Green Smoothie

(Prepping time: 10 minutes | Cooking time: 0 minutes | For 4 servings)

Ingredients

- 1 cup frozen mixed berries
- ½ cup baby spinach leaves

- 2 tablespoons fresh orange juice
- 2 tablespoons water
- 1 medium-sized, ripe banana, sliced up

How To

1. Open up the lid of your food processor.
2. Add all of the listed ingredients into the blender/food processor.
3. Blend everything well until a smooth consistency has been achieved.
4. Serve chilled!

Nutritional Values (Per Serving)

- Calories: 29
- Fat: 4g
- Carbohydrates: 54g
- Protein: 18g
- Saturated Fat: 1g
- Sodium: 64 mg
- Fiber: 10g

Hearty Banana Smoothie

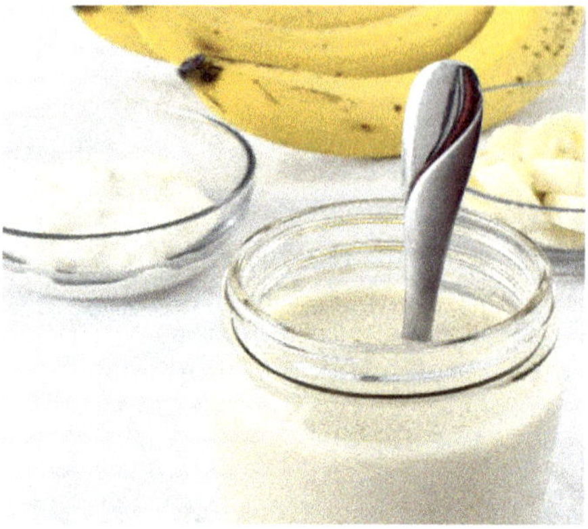

(Prepping time: 10 minutes | Cooking time: 0 minutes | For 4 servings)

Ingredients

- 1 banana
- 2 cups chopped kale
- ½ cup light, unsweetened almond milk
- 1 tablespoon flax seed

How To

1. Add the listed ingredients to your blender and blend them thoroughly.
2. Once you have a smooth mixture, chill and serve!

Nutritional Values (Per Serving)

- Calories: 311
- Fat: 7g
- Carbohydrates: 56g
- Protein: 12g

- Saturated Fat: 3g
- Sodium: 132 mg
- Fiber: 3g

Banana Strawberry Whole Wheat Muffins

(Prepping Time: 20 min. | Cooking Time: 25 mins | For 8 servings)

Ingredients

- 4 tablespoons Silk Almond milk
- 2 eggs
- 1 cup dairy-free yogurt
- 2 cups frozen strawberries, defrosted
- 2 cups mashed banana
- 1 teaspoon salt
- 3 teaspoons baking powder
- 1 teaspoon baking soda
- 2 cups whole wheat flour

How to

1. Preheat the baking oven to 325 degrees F.
2. Meanwhile, add strawberries and bananas in a bowl. Mash well.
3. Then add silk almond milk, eggs and yogurt in that bowl. Mix well until they are completely merged with each other.
4. Now, add whole wheat flour, salt, baking powder and baking soda in another bowl. Mix well.
5. Combine the two mixtures and mix properly until a smooth batter is formed.

6. Spray the muffin-tins with non-stick cooking spray and divide the batter equally in 24 muffin-tins.
7. Bake for about 25 minutes and check with a toothpick if they are completely cooked or not.
8. Take out and serve.

Nutritional Values (Per Serving)

- Calories: 193
- Fat: 1.6g
- Saturated Fat: 0.4g
- Trans Fat: 1.2g
- Carbohydrates: 39.9g
- Fiber: 2.7g
- Sodium: 483mg
- Protein: 5.7g

Plum and Strawberry Smoothie

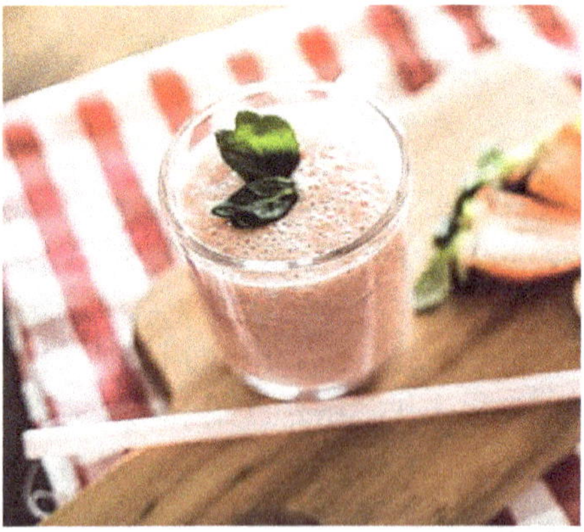

(Prepping Time: 10 min. | Cooking Time: 0 min | For 4 servings)

Ingredients

- 2 plums, pitted and chopped
- 1 cup unsweetened almond milk
- 2 cups green tea, brewed and cooled
- 4 cups frozen strawberries
- ½ cup ice cubes, crushed

How to

1. Hull the strawberries.
2. Place all the ingredients in a blender and blend until a smooth mixture is formed.
3. Pour the mixture in 4 glasses and serve.

Nutritional Values (Per Serving)

- Calories: 75
- Fat: 1g
- Saturated Fat: 0.1g
- Trans Fat: 0.8g
- Carbohydrates: 17.5g
- Fiber: 3.7g
- Sodium: 46mg
- Protein: 0.5g

Egg whites scrambled with cheese and spinach

(Prepping Time: 10 minutes | Cooking Time: 10 minutes | For 4 servings)

Ingredients

- 12 egg whites
- 8 cups baby spinach
- 4 tomatoes, chopped
- 1 cup onion, chopped
- 1 cup reduced-fat feta cheese, crumbled
- salt and pepper to taste

How to

1. Spray a non-stick skillet with cooking spray and place over medium heat.
2. Sauté the onions until translucent
3. Add the rest of the ingredients apart from the cheese and scramble. Cook until the egg white is cooked through.
4. Remove from heat and add the cheese, stirring, so it melts.
5. Season to taste and serve hot.

Nutritional Values (Per Serving)

- Calories: 179
- Fat: 4.7g
- Saturated Fat: 3.1g
- Trans Fat: 0.1g
- Carbohydrates: 11.4g
- Fiber: 3.4g
- Sodium: 474mg
- Protein: 18.9g

Hot Chocolate Mix

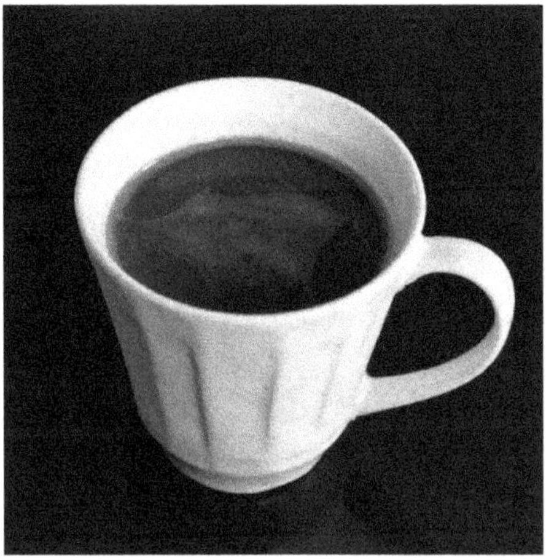

(Prepping Time: 60 minutes. | Cooking Time: 5 minutes | For 32 servings)

Ingredients

- 3 cup(s)s fat-free powdered milk
- 1 cup(s) powdered coffee creamer, vanilla flavor, sugar-free
- 1 1/3 cup(s) cocoa powder, unsweetened
- 2 tablespoon(s) cinnamon

How To

1. Put all of your ingredients in a mason jar or similar airtight container. Make sure they are thoroughly mixed.
2. To serve, put 3 tablespoon(s) in a cup(s) and top with boiling water.
3. Serve hot.

Nutritional Values (Per serving)

- Calories: 52
- Fat: 17.6g
- Saturated Fat: 1.4g
- Trans Fat: 0g
- Carbohydrates: 7.1g
- Fiber: 3.1g
- Sodium: 588mg
- Protein: 7.4g

Apple Cider

(Prepping Time: 20 minutes | Cooking Time: 10 minutes | For 24 servings)

Ingredients

- 2 large oranges
- 6 cloves
- 6 cup(s)s orange juice, unsweetened
- 4 quarts apple juice, unsweetened
- 1/2 cup(s) raisins
- 2 cinnamon sticks

How To

1. Squeeze the oranges and add their juice to the rest of the orange juice.
2. Stick the cloves into the squeezed orange cup(s)s.

3. Place all of your ingredients in in a pot over high heat.
4. Bring to a boil then remove from heat.
5. Cover and allow to rest for 30 minutes at least.
6. Serve hot.

Nutritional Values (Per Serving)

- Calories: 110
- Fat: 0.3g
- Saturated Fat: 0g
- Trans Fat: 0g
- Carbohydrates: 27g
- Fiber: 1g
- Sodium: 8mg
- Protein: 1g

Appetizers and Sides

Cinnamon Apples

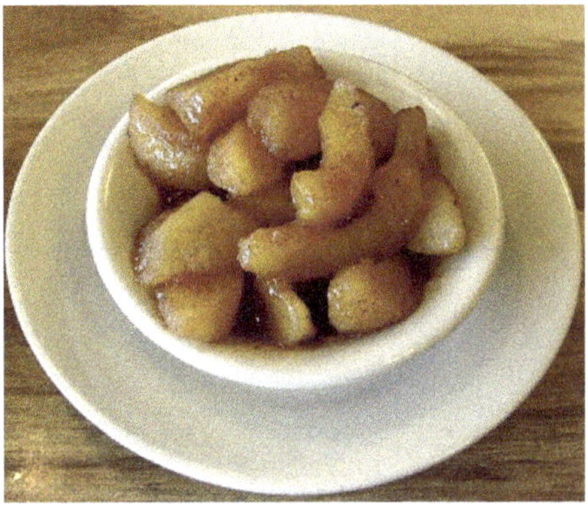

(Prepping time: 10 minutes | Cooking time: 10 minutes | For 4 servings)

Ingredients

- 1 cup of coconut oil
- ¼ cup date paste
- 2 tablespoons ground cinnamon
- 4 granny smith apples, peeled and sliced, cored

How To

1. Take a large-sized skillet and place it over medium heat
2. Add oil and allow the oil to heat up
3. Stir in cinnamon and date paste into the oil
4. Add cut up apples and cook for 5-8 minutes until crispy
5. Serve and enjoy!

Nutritional Values (Per Serving)

- Calories: 368
- Fat: 21g
- Carbohydrates: 34g
- Protein: 1g
- Saturated Fat: 3g
- Sodium: 120mg
- Fiber: 3g

Delicious Cabbage Soup

(Prepping time: 7 minutes | Cooking time: 25 minutes | For 4 servings)

Ingredients

- 3 cups non-fat beef stock
- 2 garlic cloves, minced
- 1 tablespoon of tomato paste
- 2 cup cabbage, chopped
- ½ a yellow onion
- ½ a cup carrot, chopped
- ½ a cup green beans
- ½ a cup zucchini, chopped
- ½ a teaspoon of basil
- ½ a teaspoon of oregano
- Salt and pepper as needed

How To

1. Grease a pot with nonstick cooking spray
2. Place it over medium heat and allow the oil the heat up
3. Add onions, carrots, and garlic and Sauté for 5 minutes
4. Add broth, tomato paste, green beans, cabbage, basil, oregano, salt, and pepper
5. Bring the whole mix to a boil and lower down the heat, simmer for 5-10 minutes until all veggies are tender
6. Add zucchini and simmer for 5 minutes more
7. Sever hot and enjoy!

Nutritional Values (Per Serving)

- Calories: 22
- Fat: 0g
- Carbohydrates: 5g
- Protein: 1g
- Saturated Fat: 0g
- Sodium: 759mg
- Fiber: 1g

Tuna Spread

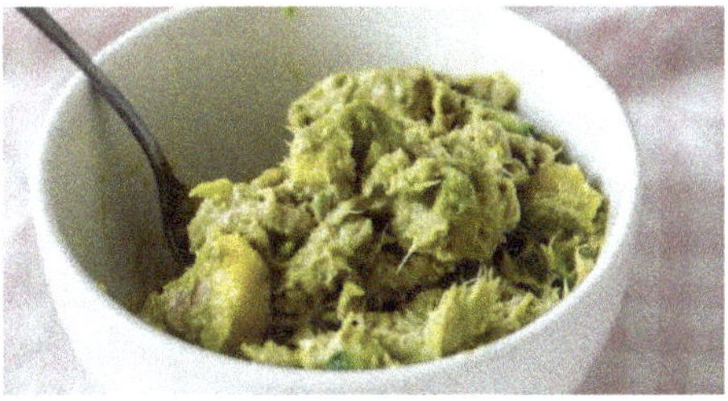

(Prepping Time: 5 minutes | Cooking Time: 15 minutes | For 20 servings)

Ingredients

- 8 oz tuna canned in water
- 4 teaspoon(s) light mayonnaise sauce
- 12 oz fat free cream cheese, softened
- 4 teaspoon(s) dill
- 1 teaspoon(s) capers
- 3 tablespoon(s) lemon juice, freshly squeezed

How To

1. Mix all of the ingredients and refrigerate overnight.

2. Serve over whole wheat bagels (calories & points for the bagels not included).

Nutritional Values (Per Serving)

- Calories: 31
- Fat: 0.6g
- Saturated Fat: 0.2g
- Trans Fat: 0g
- Carbohydrates: 2g
- Fiber: 0g
- Sodium: 158mg
- Protein: 5g

Sesame Ginger Dressing

(Prepping Time: 10 minutes | Cooking Time: 1 minute | For 32 servings)

Ingredients

- 1/4 cup(s) light soy sauce
- 3/4 cup(s) canola oil
- 1/4 cup(s) tablespoon(s) rice wine vinegar
- 1 1/2 tablespoon(s) sesame oil
- 1 1/2 tablespoon(s) lime juice
- 1 1/2 cloves of garlic, minced
- 1/4 cup(s) honey
- 1 1/2 tablespoon(s) ginger, grated
- 1 1/2 teaspoon(s) low calorie Sriracha
- 1/4 cup(s) water

How To

1. Place all the juices in a bowl and mix well to combine. Save ¼ of the marinade separately. Set aside
2. Using a mandolin slicer slice the fennel bulb into thin slices. Add it to the first bowl and mix.
3. Do the same for the artichokes, and zucchini.
4. Slice the beetroot into thin slices and add it to the second bowl.
5. Using Saran wrap, cover the bowls. Make sure the vegetables will stay under the marinade.
6. Place in the refrigerator for 12 hours
7. Arrange onto a serving platter, along with the cubed avocado.
8. Top with arugula, salt& pepper to taste, and balsamic cream.

Nutritional Values (Per Serving)

- Calories: 63
- Fat: 5.8g
- Saturated Fat: 0.5g
- Trans Fat: 0.1g
- Carbohydrates: 2.7g
- Fiber: 0g
- Sodium: 121mg
- Protein: 0.3g

Spinach Salad

(Prepping Time: 15 minutes | Cooking Time: 20 minutes | For 12 servings)

Ingredients

- 9 slices of turkey bacon
- 4 portobello mushrooms, sliced
- 2 tablespoon(s) canola oil
- 1 teaspoon(s) thyme
- 1 teaspoon(s) rosemary
- 4 1/2 tablespoon(s) balsamic vinegar
- 1 1/2 teaspoon(s) Dijon mustard
- 3/4 cup(s) canola oil
- 10 1/2 ounces baby spinach
- 1 1/2 red onion, thinly sliced

How To

1. Line a microwave-safe dish with paper towels and place the bacon on it. Microwave for 2 minutes on high. If it's not crispy microwave for a little longer.
2. Crumble and set aside.
3. In a skillet over medium-high heat, heat the oil and add the mushrooms, salt and pepper to taste, the thyme, the and rosemary. Toss gently and cook for about 6 minutes, stirring often, until the mushrooms cook and dry a little.
4. Remove from the heat and set aside. to cool.
5. Place the vinegar, the mustard, and the salt and pepper in a bowl and whisk.
6. Slowly drizzle in olive oil, while whisking.
7. Place the spinach, the onions, and the mushrooms in a salad bowl then sprinkle with the bacon.
8. Dress the salad right before you serve it.

Nutritional Values (Per Serving)

- Calories: 182
- Fat: 17.8g
- Saturated Fat: 1.6g
- Trans Fat: 0.1g
- Carbohydrates: 3g
- Fiber: 1g
- Sodium: 153g
- Protein: 3g

Salmon Spread

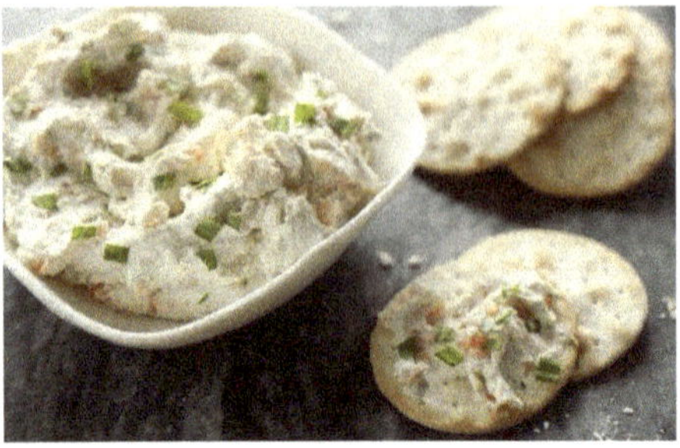

(Prepping Time: 5 minutes | Cooking Time: 15 minutes | For 20 servings)

Ingredients

- 8 oz salmon, fillets, skin removed, in chunks
- 4 teaspoon Worcestershire sauce
- 12 oz fat-free cream cheese, softened
- 4 teaspoon dill
- 3 tablespoon lemon juice, freshly squeezed

How to

1. Mix all of the ingredients and refrigerate overnight.
2. Serve over whole wheat bagels (calories not included).

Nutritional Values (Per Serving)

- Calories: 76
- Fat: 6.7g
- Saturated Fat: 3.9g
- Trans Fat: 0.1g
- Carbohydrates: 0.8
- Fiber: 0g

- Sodium: 67mg
- Protein: 3.5g

Zucchini Pie

(Prepping Time: 20 min | Cooking Time: 35 min | For 12 servings)

Ingredients

- 2 cups zucchini, chopped
- 4 eggs
- ¼ teaspoon pepper
- 2 cups tomatoes, chopped
- 1 teaspoon salt
- 1 cup onion, chopped
- 2 cups milk
- ½ cup grated Parmesan cheese
- 1 cup original Bisquick Baking Mix

How to

1. Preheat the baking oven to 400 degrees F and grease a pie dish.
2. Place zucchini, onion, tomatoes, and cheese in the pie dish.
3. Meanwhile, add milk, salt, baking mix, pepper, and eggs in a bowl and mix well. Pour into the dish.
4. Bake for about 35 minutes and insert a toothpick to check if it is completely cooked or not.
5. Take out and set aside for 5 minutes.
6. Serve and enjoy!

Nutritional Values (Per Serving)

- Calories: 98
- Fat: 4.1g
- Saturated Fat: 1.5g
- Trans Fat: 2.7g
- Carbohydrates: 10.9g
- Fiber: 1g
- Sodium: 369mg
- Protein: 4.9g

Spinach Crepes

(Prepping Time: 65 minutes | Cooking Time: 10 minutes. | For 12 servings)

Ingredients

- 4 eggs, room temperature
- 2 egg yolk
- 1 cup milk
- 3.5oz gluten-free flour
- 3.5oz spinach
- 1 tablespoon margarine 20% fat

How to

1. Put all the ingredients in a bowl and beat with a mixer until you get a smooth batter.

2. Cover the bowl with shrink wrap and chill for a minimum of 1 hour.
3. In a non-stick skillet over medium heat, melt half a tablespoon margarine.
4. Pour a ladleful of the batter in the pan and rotate to cover the bottom
5. Cook for 2 minutes and check with a spatula if the edges of the crepe lift. Flip the crepe and cook from the other side for another 2 minutes.
6. Repeat until you run out of batter.

Nutritional Values (Per Serving)

- Calories: 74
- Fat: 3g
- Saturated Fat: 1.1g
- Trans Fat: 0.1g
- Carbohydrates: 8.1g
- Fiber: 1.1g
- Sodium: 72mg
- Protein: 25.2g

Balsamic-Glazed Sprouts

(Prepping time: 10 minutes \ Cooking time: 30 minutes | For 4 servings)

Ingredients

- ½ pound Brussels sprouts, trimmed and halved
- Fresh cracked black pepper

- 1 tablespoon olive oil
- Salt to taste
- 2 teaspoons balsamic glaze
- 2 wooden skewers

How To

1. Take wooden skewers and place them on a largely sized foil
2. Place sprouts on the skewers and drizzle oil sprinkle salt and pepper
3. Cover skewers with foil
4. Preheat your grill to low and place skewers (with foil) in the grill
5. Grill for 30 minutes, making sure to turn after every 5-6 minutes
6. Once done, uncovered and drizzle balsamic glaze on top
7. Enjoy!

Nutritional Values (Per Serving)

- Calories: 400
- Fat: 27g
- Carbohydrates: 23g
- Protein: 26g
- Saturated Fat: 7g
- Sodium: 198mg
- Fiber: 2g

Toasty Guac

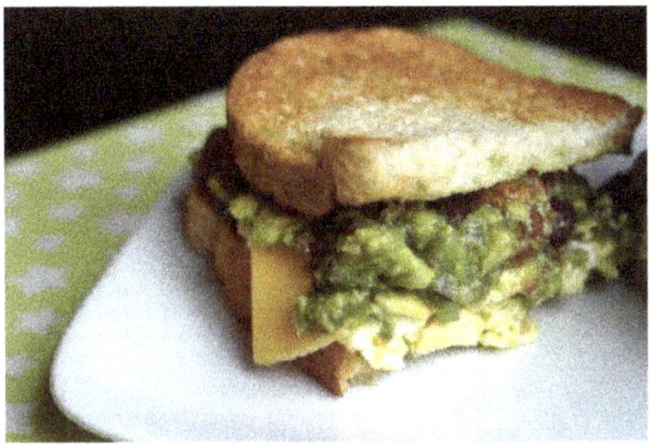

(Prepping time: 10 minutes | Cooking time: 5 minutes | For 4 servings)

Ingredients

- 1 cup beans, cooked
- 2 medium tomato, finely chopped
- ½ a medium avocado, chopped
- 1 tablespoon lime juice
- 2 tablespoons fresh coriander, chopped
- 4 slices toasted multigrain bread

How To

1. Take a small-sized bowl and add beans, tomato, lime juice, coriander, and mix
2. Season mix with salt and pepper
3. Spoon the mixture over toast
4. Serve and enjoy!

Nutritional Values (Per Serving)

- Calories: 173
- Fat: 15g
- Carbohydrates: 12g
- Protein: 2g

- Saturated Fat: 4g
- Sodium: 320mg
- Fiber: 2g

Sticky Rice Pudding

(Prepping time: 10 minutes | Cooking time: 25 minutes | For 4 Serving)

Ingredients

- 2 cups of fat-free Milk
- ¼ cup of sugar
- 2 tablespoon of water
- 1 and a 1/3 cup of Arborio rice
- 2 large eggs
- ¼ cup of golden raisins
- 1 teaspoon of vanilla extract
- Pinch of cinnamon
- 4 teaspoon of butter

How To

1. Add 1 cup of Milk, sugar, water to a small saucepan
2. Bring to mix to a boil
3. Stir in rice and lower down the heat to low, simmer for 30 minutes making sure to keep stirring it from time to time
4. Preheat your Oven to 325 degrees Fahrenheit
5. Spray 1 and a ½ quart baking dish with nonstick cooking spray
6. Add 1 cup of Milk, eggs, vanilla, raisins, and cinnamon to a medium bowl
7. Stir in rice
8. Pour the mix into a baking dish and dot with butter
9. Bake for 25 minutes
10. Enjoy!

Nutritional Values (Per Serving)

- Calories: 238
- Fat: 2 g
- Saturated Fat: 1 g
- Carbohydrates: 40 g
- Fiber: 3 g
- Sodium: 84 mg
- Protein: 7 g

Ranch Dressing

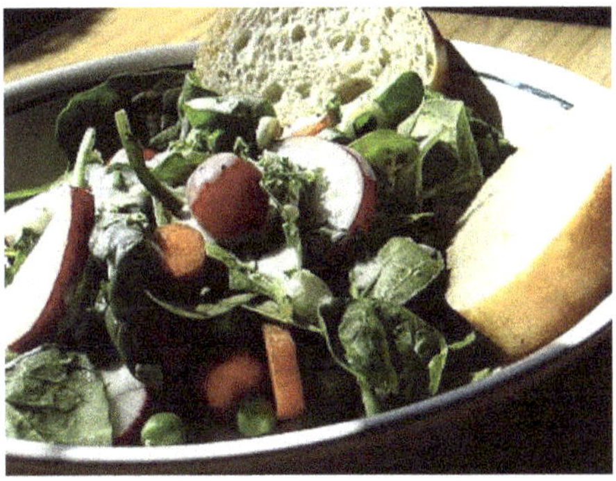

(Prep Time: 10 minutes | Cooking Time: 10 minutes | For 64 Servings)

Ingredients

- 1 3/4 cup(s) coconut milk, unsweetened
- 1 3/4 cup(s) light mayonnaise
- 2/3 cup(s) vinegar
- 2 2/3 tablespoon(s) parsley, chopped
- 1 3/4 tablespoon(s) basil, chopped
- 1 3/4 tablespoon(s) thyme, chopped
- 3/4 tablespoon(s) peppermint, chopped

- 1 3/4 tablespoon(s) dill, chopped
- 1 3/4 tablespoon(s) cilantro, chopped
- 1 3/4 tablespoon(s) oregano, chopped
- 3 1/2 cloves garlic, minced
- 3 1/2 teaspoon(s) onion, chopped
- salt and pepper to taste

How To

1. Add all of your ingredients in a blender and pulse until combined and you have reached the desired consistency.
2. Taste and add salt and pepper if needed.
3. If the dressing is too thick you can add more coconut milk to thin it.
4. Allow to chill for at least 1 hour before serving. The longer it sits the better the taste will become.

Nutritional Values (Per Serving)

- Calories: 40
- Fat: 3.7g
- Saturated Fat: 1.7g
- Trans Fat: 0g
- Carbohydrates: 2g
- Fiber: 0g
- Sodium: 48mg
- Protein: 0g

Artichoke and Hearts of Palm Salad

(Prepping Time: 10 mins | Cooking Time: 1 minutes | For 8 Servings)

Ingredients

- 3 oz Capers, rinsed
- 13 oz hearts of Palm, diced
- 13 oz artichoke hearts, halved
- 1 avocado, pitted
- 1 1/2 tablespoon(s) light mayonnaise
- 1 tablespoon(s) lemon juice

How To

For the bread:

1. Mix the lemon juice with the mayonnaise.
2. Mix the rest of your ingredients together in a bowl and combine with the dressing.
3. Serve cold.

Nutritional Values (Per Serving)

- Calories: 127
- Fat: 4.9g
- Saturated Fat: 0.7g
- Trans Fat: 0g
- Carbohydrates: 20g
- Fiber: 5g
- Sodium: 321mg
- Protein: 4g

Turmeric Energy Bites

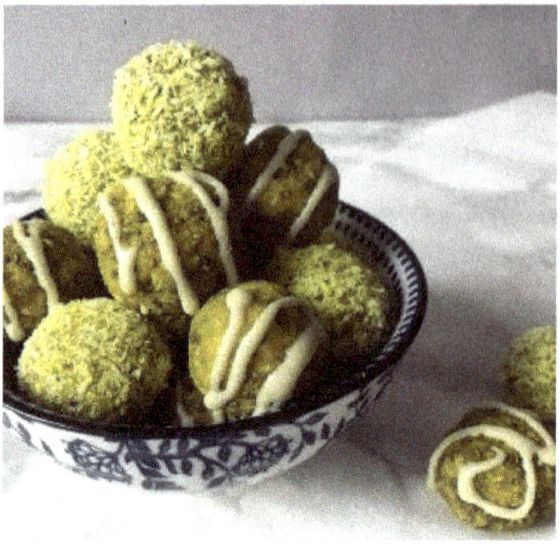

(Prepping Time: 15 min. | Cooking Time: 0 min | For 8 Servings)

Ingredients

- 3 teaspoons turmeric powder
- 2 teaspoons coconut oil
- 2 cups almond butter
- 1 cup unsweetened coconut flakes
- 1 teaspoon maple syrup
- 1 teaspoon honey

How To

1. Add turmeric powder, honey, maple syrup, almond butter, and coconut oil in a blender and blend well.
2. Take out and make small balls out of the mixture.
3. Roll all the balls in coconut flakes before serving.
4. Enjoy!

Nutritional Values (Per Serving)

- Calories: 77
- Fat: 6.5g
- Saturated Fat: 3.7g
- Trans Fat: 2.2g
- Carbohydrates: 4.6g
- Fiber: 1.6g
- Sodium: 1mg
- Protein: 1.4g

Blackberry Leather

(Prepping Time: 30 min | Cooking Time: 6 hours | For 10 Servings)

Ingredients

- ½ cup unsweetened applesauce
- ½ teaspoon fresh lemon juice
- 4 cups fresh blackberries
- 2 teaspoons ground cinnamon
- ½ teaspoon maple syrup
- 2 tablespoons fresh mint leaves, chopped

How To

1. Line a baking sheet with parchment paper and preheat the oven to 170 degrees F.
2. Meanwhile, add all the ingredients in a blender and pulse until smooth.
3. Pour the mixture on the baking sheet and spread it with the top of spoon.
4. Bake for 6 hours and take out.

5. With the help of knife, cut the leather into rectangular pieces.
6. Roll those rectangles and serve.

Nutritional Values (Per Serving)

- Calories: 33
- Fat: 0.3g
- Saturated Fat: 0g
- Trans Fat: 0.2g
- Carbohydrates: 7.6g
- Fiber: 3.5g
- Sodium: 1mg
- Protein: 0.9g

Pomegranate Salad Dressing

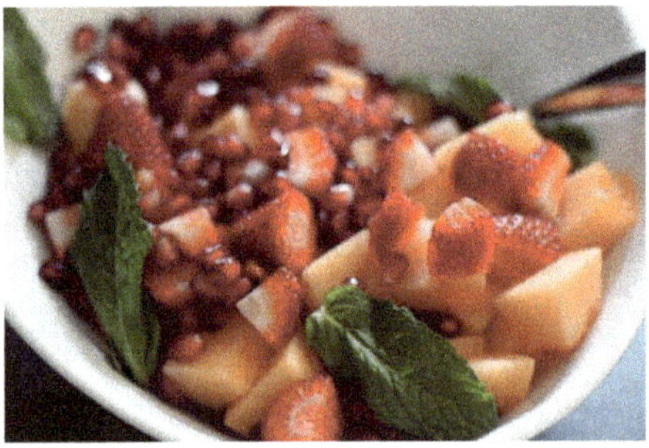

(Prepping Time: 10 minutes | Cooking Time: 2 minutes | For 64 Servings)

Ingredients

- 4 teaspoons thyme
- 4 tablespoon marjoram
- 4 tablespoon basil
- 4 teaspoons lemon zest
- 4 teaspoons orange zest

- 1/2 cup sugar-free maple syrup
- 1/2 cup mustard
- 1 cup sherry vinegar
- 4 pints sugar-free pomegranate juice

How To

1. Pour all ingredients into a blender.
2. Mix until everything is well combined
3. Store in the fridge and serve over a salad

Nutritional Values (Per Serving-3 tablespoon)

- Calories: 13
- Fat: 0g
- Saturated Fat: 0g
- Trans Fat: 0g
- Carbohydrates: 0.6g
- Fiber: 0.3g
- Sodium: 21mg
- Protein: 0.1g

Baked Omelet

(Prepping Time: 10 minutes | Cooking Time: 30 minutes | For 4 Servings)

Ingredients

- 6 eggs
- salt and pepper
- 1 tomato, diced
- 1 green bell pepper, diced
- 2oz fat-free parmesan cheese, grated

- 1 tablespoon margarine 20% fat, melted

How To

1. Preheat oven to 350F.
2. Spray a 6-inch round baking dish with cooking spray
3. In a bowl, crack the eggs and add salt and pepper to taste. Whisk well.
4. Add the peppers, parmesan, and tomatoes to the bowl—season to taste.
5. Pour the mixture into the Preppingared dish and drizzle with the melted margarine.
6. Bake for 15 minutes until the omelet is firm
7. Serve immediately.

Nutritional Values (Per Serving)

- Calories: 298
- Fat: 9.9g
- Saturated Fat: 3.7g
- Trans Fat: 0g
- Carbohydrates: 23.4g
- Fiber: 0.6g
- Sodium: 256mg
- Protein: 28.7g

Pumpkin Pie Oatmeal

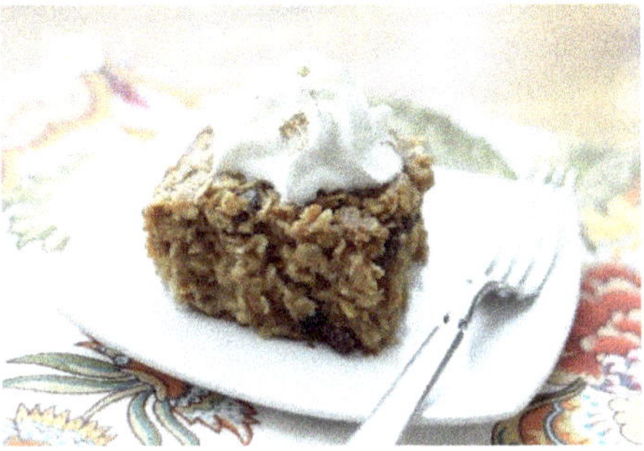

(Prepping time: 10 minutes | Cooking time: 10 minutes | For 4 servings)

Ingredients

- ½ cup canned pumpkin
- Mashed banana as needed
- ¾ cup unsweetened almond milk
- ½ teaspoon pumpkin pie spice
- 1 cup oats
- 2 teaspoons maple syrup

How To

1. Mash banana using fork and mix in the remaining ingredients (except oats) and mix well
2. Add oats and finely stir
3. Transfer mixture to a pot and let the oats cook until it has absorbed the liquid and are tender
4. Serve and enjoy!

Nutritional Values (Per Serving)

- Calories: 264

- Fat: 4g
- Carbohydrates: 34g
- Protein: 7g
- Saturated Fat: 1g
- Sodium: 246mg
- Fiber: 4g

Chicken And Parm Cutlet

(Prepping time: 10 minutes | Cooking time: 25 minutes | For 4 servings)

Ingredients

- 4 chicken breasts, boneless
- ¼ teaspoon pepper
- ½ teaspoon garlic powder
- 1 teaspoon dried parsley
- 1/8 teaspoon paprika
- 2 tablespoon seasoned Italian crumbs
- ¼ cup parmesan cheese, grated

How To

1. Preheat your Oven to a temperature of 400-degree Fahrenheit
2. Take a resealable plastic bag and combine cheese, seasoning, and crumbs
3. Shake everything well
4. Transfer the mix to a bowl and dip your chicken breast in the cheese mix, making sure to turn the breast well to coat both sides

5. Take a nonstick baking sheet and arrange the seasoned breasts on top
6. Bake the chicken for about 25 minutes in your oven until it is cooked thoroughly
7. Serve hot!

Nutritional Values (Per Serving)

- Calories: 669
- Fat: 43g
- Carbohydrates: 36g
- Protein: 34g
- Saturated Fat: 13g
- Sodium: 335mg
- Fiber: 2g

Butternut Squash Bake

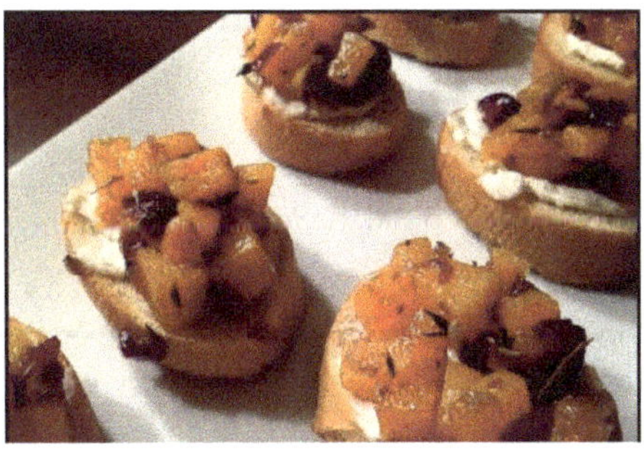

(Prepping Time: 15 minutes | Cooking Time: 30 | For 6 servings)

Ingredients

- 6 cup(s)s Butternut Squash, peeled and diced
- 1/2 cup(s) granulated sugar
- 2 tablespoon(s) low-fat margarine
- 1/4 teaspoon(s) cinnamon

How To

1. Melt the butter and mix with the sugar and the cinnamon in a bowl.
2. Place the squash in the bowl and toss to get it covered.
3. Transfer to a baking dish and bake at 400F for 30 minutes.
4. Serve warm.

Nutritional Values (Per Serving)

- Calories: 129
- Fat: 3.9g
- Saturated Fat: 0.7g
- Trans Fat: 0g
- Carbohydrates: 25g
- Fiber: 3g
- Sodium: 7mg
- Protein: 1g

Kale Crepes

(Prepping Time: 65 minutes | Cooking Time: 10 minutes. | For 8 crepes)

Ingredients

- 3 large eggs, room temperature
- 1 large egg yolk
- 2/3 cup(s) fat free milk
- 2/3 tablespoon(s) low-fat margarine
- 2 1/3 oz flour
- 2 1/3 oz Kale

How To

1. Add all of the ingredients in a bowl and mix until smooth.
2. Cover the bowl with Saran wrap and chill for at least 1 hour.
3. In a non-stick pan over medium heat melt half a tablespoon(s) margarine.
4. Take a ladle and pour some of the batter in the pan. Rotate to cover the bottom.
5. Cook for 2 minutes then check if the edges of the crepe can be lifted.
6. Flip the crepe and cook the other side for another 2 minutes.
7. Repeat until you finish with the batter.

Nutritional Values (Per Serving)

- Calories: 79
- Fat: 3.3g
- Saturated Fat: 1.2g
- Trans Fat: 0g
- Carbohydrates: 8g
- Fiber: 1g
- Sodium: 43mg
- Protein: 4g

Cheese and Onion Poppers

(Prepping Time: 10 minutes | Cooking Time: 10 minutes | For 24 servings)

Ingredients

- 2 1/3 cup(s)s light biscuit mix
- 3/4 cup(s) nonfat milk
- 2/3 cup(s) low fat Cheddar cheese, shredded
- 1/3 cup(s) green onions, sliced
- 2 1/3 tablespoon(s) 20% margarine, melted

How To

1. Preheat your oven to 450F.
2. Spray a baking sheet with non-stick spray.
3. In a large bowl, add the biscuit mix the, milk, the cheese, and the onions. Mix until you form a dough.
4. Use a teaspoon(s) to dollop balls of dough on the Preppingared sheet
5. Bake for about 8 minutes, until golden brown.
6. Brush with the melted margarine when warm.
7. Serve with the dip of your liking. (Calories and points not included).

Nutritional Values (Per Serving)

- Calories: 97
- Fat: 2.1g
- Saturated Fat: 0.2g
- Trans Fat: 0g
- Carbohydrates: 3.7g
- Fiber: 3.2g

- Sodium: 283mg
- Protein: 16.6g

Cashew Cream

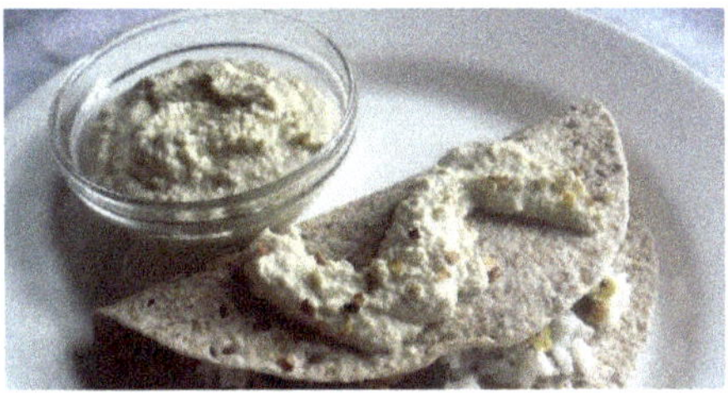

(Prepping Time: 5 minutes | Cooking Time: 65 minutes | For 12 servings)

Ingredients

- 1 cup+2 tablespoon cashews
- ⅔ cup of water
- 1 teaspoon salt

How to

1. Put the cashews in a bowl and cover with water. Soak for 1 hour.
2. Drain (save ⅔ cup of the water) and put in a food processor along with the soaking water you saved.
3. Add the salt and blend until creamy.

Nutritional Values (Per Serving)

- Calories: 23

- Fat: 1.8g
- Saturated Fat: 0.3g
- Trans Fat: 0g
- Carbohydrates: 1g
- Fiber: 0.1g
- Sodium: 195mg
- Protein: 0.7g

Stuffed Mushrooms

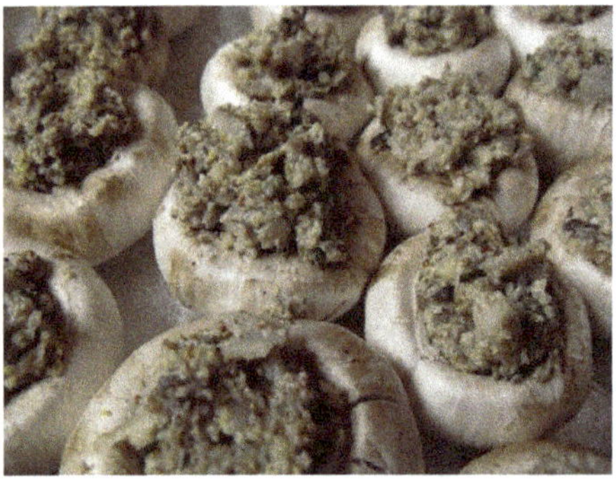

(Prepping Time: 10 min | Cooking Time: 10 min | For 2 servings)

Ingredients

- 4 mushrooms, stemmed
- ½ shallot, chopped
- 1 tablespoon grated Pecorino cheese
  ½ garlic clove
- 2 tablespoons non-fat cottage cheese
- ½ tablespoon olive oil

- 1 small sun-dried tomato, chopped
- 1 cup small spinach leaves, chopped

How to

1. Heat the baking oven to 350 degrees F and grease the baking dish.
2. Add shallot, garlic, and mushrooms in a processor and pulse well.
3. Now, add oil and shallot mixture in a skillet and stir properly on low flame.
4. Add in tomato and cook for 5 more minutes.
5. Then add spinach and stir well until it wilts.
6. Take out in a bowl and add in cottage cheese and pecorino cheese.
7. Fill the mixture in the mushrooms and place them on the baking dish.
8. Bake for 10 to 12 minutes and take out.
9. Serve hot.

Nutritional Values (Per Serving)

- Calories: 70
- Fat: 4.9g
- Saturated Fat: 1g
- Trans Fat: 3.9g
- Carbohydrates: 3.2g
- Fiber: 0.8g
- Sodium: 136mg
- Protein: 4.6g

Guacamole

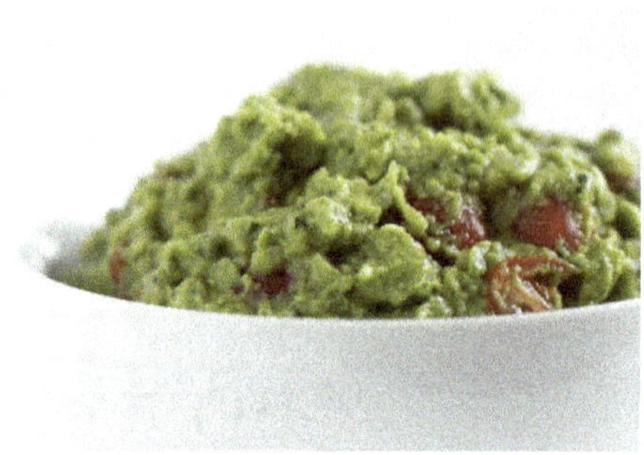

(Prepping Time: 15 minutes | Cooking Time: - | For 3 pints)

Ingredients

- 4 cups peas, cooked, rinsed, and drained
- 4 medium avocados, peeled and pitted, mashed
- Juice of 4 limes
- 2 teaspoons salt
- 2 cups tomatoes, diced
- 2 cups onion, diced
- 1 cup parsley, finely chopped
- 4 jalapeños, seeded and minced
- 8 cloves of garlic, minced

How to

1. In a high-speed blender, pulse the peas until smooth.
2. Add the rest of the ingredients apart from the avocado and pulse again until they're combined but still a little chunky.
3. Add the avocado and stir it in with a fork.
4. Serve with vegetable sticks or nachos (calories not included)

Nutritional Values (Per Serving)

- Calories: 92
- Fat: 7g
- Saturated Fat: 1.3g
- Trans Fat: 0g
- Carbohydrates: 9.1g
- Fiber: 5g
- Sodium: 201mg
- Protein: 2.4g

Lunch and Dinner

Balsamic Chicken And Berries

(Prepping time: 10 minutes | Cooking time: 20 minutes | For 4 servings)

Ingredients

- 3 chicken breasts, skinless and boneless
- Salt as needed
- Black pepper as needed
- ¼ cup all-purpose flour
- 2/3 cup low-fat chicken broth
- 1 ½ teaspoon corn starch
- ½ cup low-sugar raspberry preserve
- 1 ½ tablespoon balsamic vinegar

How To

1. Cut the chicken into bite-sized pieces and season with salt and pepper.
2. Dredge the meat into flour and shake off excess.
3. Take a nonstick skillet and place it over medium heat.
4. Add chicken and cook for 15 minutes, turning once halfway through.
5. Remove cooked chicken and transfer to a plate.
6. Add cornstarch, chicken broth, and raspberry preserve to the skillet, then
7. stir in balsamic vinegar. Keep the heat on medium.
8. Transfer the cooked chicken to the skillet.
9. Cook for 15 minutes more, making sure to turn once.

10. Serve and enjoy!

Nutritional Values (Per Serving)

- Calories: 546
- Fat: 35g
- Carbohydrates: 11g
- Protein: 44g
- Saturated Fat: 7g
- Sodium: 228 mg
- Fiber: 10g

Super Lemon Chicken

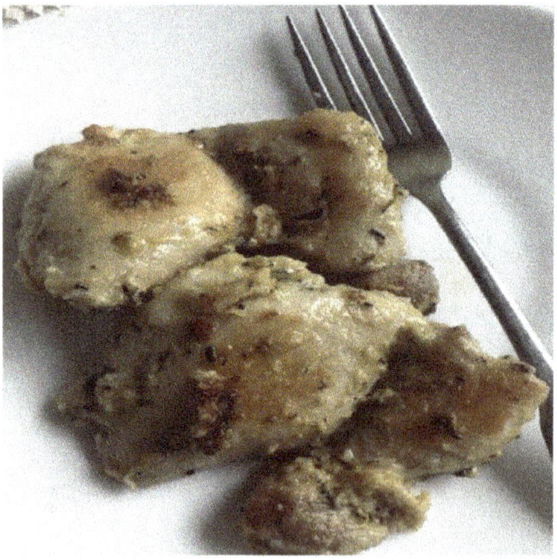

(Prepping time: 10 minutes | Cooking time: 20 minutes | For 4 servings)

Ingredients

- 1 ¼ pounds chicken breast, boneless and skinless

- 2 tablespoons almond flour
- 1 teaspoon garlic powder
- ½ teaspoon pepper
- ½ teaspoon of salt
- 1 lemon
- 1 tablespoon olive oil
- 2 cups chopped asparagus
- 2 minced cloves garlic
- ½ cup low-sodium chicken broth
- 1 tablespoon white wine vinegar

How To

1. Combine flour, garlic powder, lemon zest, pepper, and salt.
2. Toss the chicken with the mixture until the pieces are coated.
3. Place a medium-sized skillet over medium heat.
4. Add olive oil and heat it up, then add the chicken and cook on each side
5. for 2-3 minutes until browned.
6. Remove the browned chicken and keep It on the side
7. Add asparagus and garlic to the skillet and cook for 2-3 minutes.
8. Add chicken broth and vinegar to the skillet.
9. Stir and scrape the browned bits.
10. Transfer the browned chicken back and allow it to simmer for 5-10 minutes on low heat.
11. Squeeze lemon juice on top.
12. Enjoy!

Nutritional Values (Per Serving)

- Calories: 239
- Fat: 5g
- Carbohydrates: 10g

- Protein: 38g
- Saturated Fat: 2g
- Sodium: 257 mg
- Fiber: 2g

Salisbury Steak

(Prepping time: 10 minutes | Cooking time: 10 minutes | For 4 servings)

Ingredients

- 1 pound ground beef, extra lean
- ¼ teaspoon garlic powder
- ½ teaspoon kosher salt
- ¼ teaspoon black pepper
- 8 ounces mushrooms, sliced
- ¼ cup onion, minced
- 1 teaspoon dried thyme
- 2 tablespoons dry sherry or White Wine
- 12 ounces fat-free beef gravy

How To

1. Place ground beef in a small bowl, season with salt and pepper, and mix.
2. Shape the mix into 4 half-inch-thick patties.
3. Grease a large nonstick skillet with cooking spray.
4. Place it over medium-high heat and allow it to heat up.
5. Add the patties to the skillet and cook for 4 minutes per side.
6. Remove patties from the skillet and set them aside.

7. Increase the heat to medium-high and add onion, mushrooms, and
8. thyme. Sauté for 3 minutes.
9. Add sherry and sauté for 1 minute more.
10. Add gravy and return the cooked patties to the skillet.
11. Cook for 2 minutes more and enjoy!

Nutritional Values (Per Serving)

- Calories: 225
- Fat: 8g
- Carbohydrates: 8g
- Protein: 29g
- Saturated Fat: 3g
- Sodium: 358 mg
- Fiber: 2g

Caramelized Pork Chops

(Prepping time: 10 minutes | Cooking time: 40 minutes | For 4 servings)

Ingredients

- 2 teaspoons garlic, chopped
- ½ teaspoon rosemary, dried
- 3 medium onion, sliced
- 12 teaspoons pepper
- 4 pork chops, ½ inch thick
- ¼ cup butter

How To

1. Take a 12-inch skillet and place it over medium heat
2. Add butter and allow the butter to melt until sizzling
3. Add pork chops and cook them for 8-10 minutes (covered), making sure to turn them once
4. Once they are browned, season with pepper and salt and transfer to a serving platter
5. Add the onions to your skillet (with pan juice) and garnish with rosemary
6. Cook on medium for about 8-10 minutes, stirring occasionally
7. Stir in garlic, cook for 2-3 minutes until tender
8. Return your pork chops and cook for 4-5 minutes until the chops are well cooked and no longer pink
9. Serve in your platter and enjoy!

Nutritional Values (Per Serving)

- Calories: 412
- Fat: 24g
- Carbohydrates: 2g
- Protein: 44g
- Saturated Fat: 9g
- Sodium: 211mg
- Fiber: 0g

Zucchini and Feta Bake

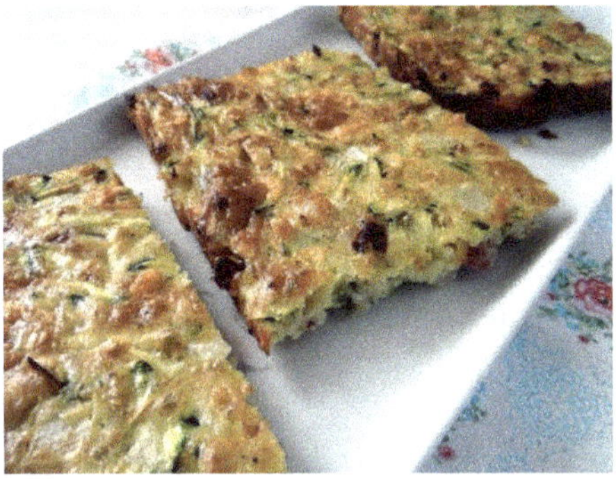

(Prepping Time: 30 minutes | Cooking Time: 40 minutes | For 8 servings)

Ingredients

- 1 tablespoon(s) olive oil
- 2 large zucchinis, diced
- 1 large onion, diced
- 1/2 teaspoon(s) oregano
- Salt and pepper to taste
- 3 large eggs
- 1 teaspoon(s) baking powder
- 1/2 cup(s) low fat plain yogurt
- 1/2 cup(s) all-purpose flour
- 8oz feta cheese, crumbled
- 2 tablespoon(s) fresh parsley, minced
- 1 teaspoon(s) paprika

How To

1. Preheat your oven to 350F
2. Heat the olive oil in a large pot over medium-high heat.
3. Add the onions, the zucchini the oregano.

4. Cook for about 10 minutes until the zucchini is tender stirring often.
5. Season with salt and pepper then remove from heat and allow to slightly cool
6. Mix the eggs and baking powder in a bowl until combined.
7. Add in the yogurt and flour and whisk to combine.
8. Add the cheese, the parsley, and the cooked veggies.
9. Grease an 8x8" baking dish.
    i. Empty the mixture into the baking dish and season with the paprika.
    ii. Bake uncovered until golden brown, around 30 minutes.
    iii. Allow to rest for 10 minutes before serving.

Nutritional Values (Per Serving)

- Calories: 159
- Fat: 9.8g
- Saturated Fat: 5.3g
- Trans Fat: 0g
- Carbohydrates: 11g
- Fiber: 1g
- Sodium: 276mg
- Protein: 7g

Stir Fry

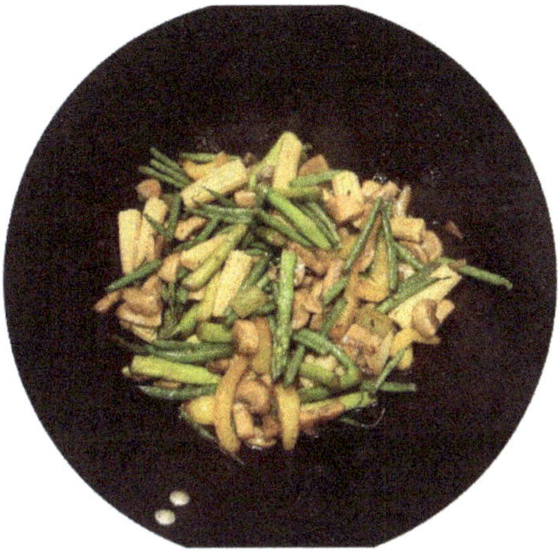

(Prepping Time: 15 minutes | Cooking Time: 15 minutes | For 12 servings)

Ingredients

- 3 cup(s)s green beans
- 1 1/2 cup(s) broccoli florets, chopped
- 3 onions
- 3 cup(s)s mushrooms, sliced
- 6 cloves of garlic, minced
- 1 1/2 cup(s) green peppers, chopped
- 9 tablespoon(s) ginger sweet and sour sauce
- 4 cup(s)s brown rice, cooked
- 1 teaspoon(s) canola oil

How To

1. Heat the oil in a wok over high heat then add the green beans, the broccoli, the onions, and the green peppers. Cook for 5 minutes stirring often.

2. Add the mushrooms, and the garlic. Cook for 5 minutes stirring often.
   Add the dressing and cook for 3 mins stirring often.
3. Remove from heat and add the rice. Mix well.
4. Serve hot.

Nutritional Values (Per Serving)

- Calories: 279
- Fat: 2.3g
- Saturated Fat: 0.4g
- Trans Fat: 0g
- Carbohydrates: 59g
- Fiber: 4g
- Sodium: 60mg
- Protein: 6g

Eggplant Bake

(Prepping Time: 15 minutes | Cooking Time: 25 minutes | For 16 servings)

Ingredients

- 3 large eggplants
- ½ cup(s) canola oil
- 3/4 cup(s) shredded low fat Swiss cheese
- 3/4 teaspoon(s) smoked paprika
- 1 ¾ teaspoon(s) garlic powder

- 1/3 teaspoon(s) dried basil
- 1/3 teaspoon(s) dried oregano
- 1/8 teaspoon(s) dried rosemary
- 1/3 teaspoon(s) dried parsley
- 1/8 teaspoon(s) dried thyme
- 1/8 teaspoon(s) red chili flakes

How To

1. Preheat your oven at 400F
2. Wash the eggplants and cut off the stem.
3. Slice the eggplants into 1/2" wheels. Put in a strainer and salt. Allow to drain for 30 minutes
4. Mix the spices the Swiss cheese and the oil in a bowl.
5. Place the eggplant in a baking dish then pour the spices mixture over them.
6. Gently toss to coat then bake for 25 minutes, flipping halfway through.
7. Serve warm.

Nutritional Values (Per Serving)

- Calories: 99
- Fat: 7.3g
- Saturated Fat: 0.7g
- Trans Fat: 0g
- Carbohydrates: 7g
- Fiber: 3g
- Sodium: 15mg
- Protein: 3g

Roasted Veggie wraps

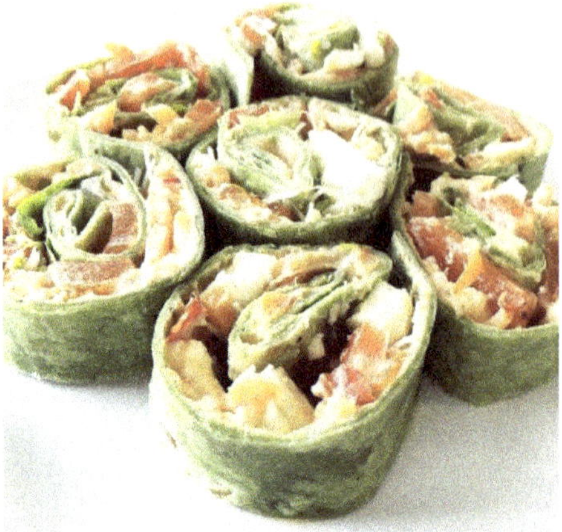

(Prepping Time: 10 minutes | Cooking Time: 40 mins | For 12 servings)

Ingredients

- 7 oz beetroots
- salt and pepper
- 1 avocado, sliced
- 6 tablespoons canola oil
- 4 cloves of garlic
- 2 tablespoon thyme
- 2 teaspoon white vinegar
- 1 cup low fat cream cheese
    - oz smoked salmon
- 7 oz arugula
- 1 dose Spinach Crepes

How to

1. Preppingare 1 dose Spinach Crepes

2. Preheat oven to 350F.
3. Scrub the beetroots and season with salt and pepper, and rubbing them lightly with canola oil, thyme, and garlic. Wrap in tinfoil bake them 40 minutes until soft
4. Peel the beets by rubbing them with paper towels. If they don't peel, they need to cook longer.
5. Grate with a box grater and put it in a bowl.
6. Add 2 tablespoons of canola oil, salt and pepper to taste, and vinegar and mix well to combine
7. Divide the cream cheese, salmon, avocado slices, arugula, and the beets mixture among the crepes, season to taste, then wrap and serve.

Nutritional Values (Per Serving)

- Calories: 291
- Fat: 17g
- Saturated Fat: 3.2g
- Trans Fat: 0.1g
- Carbohydrates: 13.6g
- Fiber: 3g
- Sodium: 785mg
- Protein: 42.8g

Tomato Cabbage Sandwich

(Prepping Time: 5 min | Cooking Time: 0 min | For 1 servings)

Ingredients

- ½ cup grated cabbage
- ½ medium tomato, sliced
- 1/8 cup thinly sliced onion
- 2 whole-wheat bread slices
- 2 romaine lettuce leaves, chopped
- 1 tablespoon Dijon mustard
- ¼ teaspoon salt
- ½ teaspoon pepper

How to

1. In a bowl, add onion, cabbage, tomato, and lettuce leaves. Stir well.
2. Now, add Dijon mustard, salt, and pepper and mix properly.
3. Place the mixture on the toasted bread slice.
4. Cover the mixture with the other bread slice and serve.

Nutritional Values (Per Serving)

- Calories: 89
- Fat: 1.4g
- Saturated Fat: 0.3g
- Trans Fat: 0.9g
- Carbohydrates: 15.4g
- Fiber: 517g
- Sodium: 654mg
- Protein: 4.6g

Broccoli-Lemon Chicken

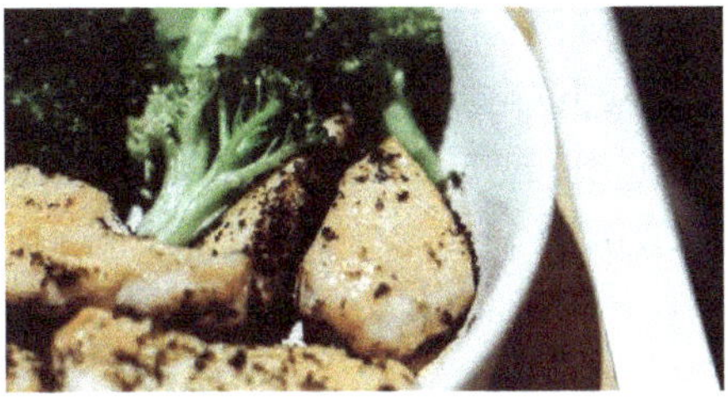

(Prepping Time: 10 min | Cooking Time: 15 min | For 8 servings)

Ingredients

- 4 tablespoons all-purpose flour
- 4 teaspoons minced garlic
- 5 cups chopped broccoli
- 2 teaspoons lemon zest
- 1 ½ pounds thinly sliced chicken breasts, boneless and skinless
- 4 tablespoons fresh parsley, chopped
- 4 teaspoons olive oil
- 2 tablespoons fresh lemon juice
- 3 cups fat-free chicken broth
- Salt and pepper, to taste

How to

1. Add 3 tablespoons flour, chicken, salt, and pepper in a bowl. Toss to coat well.
2. Meanwhile, add oil in a large skillet and heat over medium-high heat.
3. Now, add chicken in the skillet and cook for about 5 minutes.
4. Add in 2 cups broth and garlic and boil over high heat.

5. After that, add in broccoli and cook for 1 minute
6. Meanwhile, add 1 cup broth, remaining flour, and salt in a bowl and stir well.
7. Take out the chicken and add the broth mixture in the same skillet and let it simmer over low heat.
8. Cook for about 2 minutes until the mixture in skillet is slightly thick and add in chicken and lemon zest. Stir well.
9. Take out and add in parsley and lemon juice. Serve hot.

Nutritional Values (Per Serving)

- Calories: 234
- Fat: 9.4g
- Saturated Fat: 2.3g
- Trans Fat: 4.1g
- Carbohydrates: 7.9g
- Fiber: 1.7g
- Sodium: 400mg
- Protein: 28.6g

Salmon Soup

(Prepping Time: 17 min | Cooking Time: 30 min | For 10 servings)

Ingredients

- 8 cups chicken broth
- 2 tablespoons olive oil
- 2 tablespoons tamari
- 2 pounds boneless salmon

- 4 tablespoons vinegar
- 4 tablespoons chopped parsley
- Salt and black pepper, to taste

How to

1. In a large soup pan, add salmon and oil and sauté for about 5 minutes.
2. Add chicken broth and boil over high heat.
3. Lower the heat and simmer for about 15 minutes.
4. Then, add salt, pepper, vinegar and tamari and cook for 4 more minutes.
5. Take out and top it with chopped parsley.
6. Serve and enjoy!

Nutritional Values (Per Serving)

- Calories: 90
- Fat: 5.3g
- Saturated Fat: 1g
- Trans Fat: 1.9g
- Carbohydrates: 1.1g
- Fiber: 0.1g
- Sodium: 908mg
- Protein: 8.9g

Ginger Cod

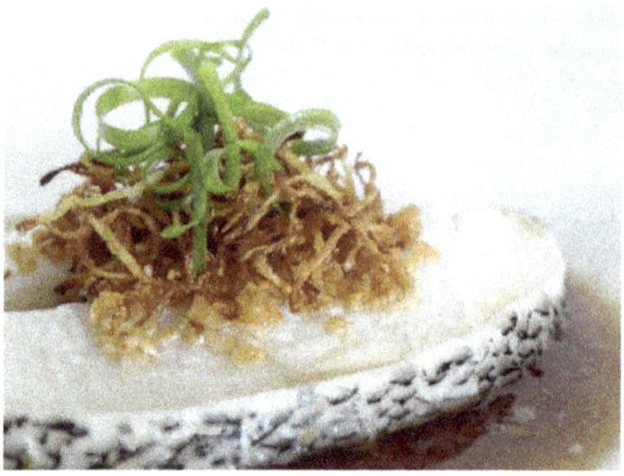

(Prepping Time: 15 min | Cooking Time: 20 min | For 8 servings)

Ingredients

- 2 pounds cod fillets
- 4 tablespoons coconut aminos
- 4 tablespoons fresh lime juice
- 2 tablespoons fresh ginger, minced
- Salt and black pepper, to taste

How to

1. Preheat the baking oven to325 degrees F and line a baking sheet with parchment paper.
2. Meanwhile, add all the ingredients except cod in a large bowl. Mix well.
3. Then add cod in the mixture and marinate it.
4. Set aside for 3 minutes and place the fillets on the baking sheet.
5. Bake for about 20 minutes and take out.
6. Serve hot.

Nutritional Values (Per Serving)

- Calories: 109
- Fat: 1.1g
- Saturated Fat: 0g
- Trans Fat: 0.5g
- Carbohydrates: 4.3g
- Fiber: 0.3g
- Sodium: 100mg
- Protein: 20.5g

Veggie Crepes

(Prepping Time: 5 minutes | Cooking Time: 10 minutes (+extra for the crepes according to the recipe) | For 12 servings)

Ingredients

- 1 dose Spinach Crepes
- 2 yellow bell pepper
- 2 green bell pepper
- 2 red bell pepper
- 6 cups sliced mushrooms
- 4 carrots, sliced
- 1 onion, thinly sliced
- 2 tablespoons olive oil
- salt and pepper to taste
- 2 cups low fat yogurt
- 1/2 bunch dill finely chopped

- Zest of 1 lemon

How to

1. Preppingare the crepes according to the recipe.
2. Slice the vegetables into 2/5-inch-thick slices and place them in a bowl. Add the oil, season to taste, and mix well.
3. Place a skillet over medium heat and sauté the vegetable mix in batches, around 4 minutes per batch until the veggies become golden.
4. In a separate bowl, mix the yogurt with the lemon zest, the dill, and season to taste.
5. Spread 2 tablespoons of yogurt in each crepe and divide the sautéed veggies among them.

Nutritional Values (Per Serving)

- Calories: 138
- Fat: 3.7g
- Saturated Fat: 1.5g
- Trans Fat: 0.1g
- Carbohydrates: 18.7g
- Fiber: 3.3g
- Sodium: 140mg
- Protein: 30.7g

Stuffed Salmon Fillets

(Prepping Time: 15 mins | Cooking Time: 20 mins | For 12 servings)

Ingredients

- 4 pounds salmon fillets
- 2 cups kale
- 8 cloves of garlic, finely chopped
- 8 tablespoons raisins
- 4 teaspoons lemon zest
- *For the crust:*
- 4 tablespoons mustard
- 2 cups panko bread crumbs

How to

1. Preheat oven to 375F.
2. Make an incision on your fillets and cut a pocket
3. Drizzle half a teaspoon of olive oil in a saucepan over medium-high heat.
4. Add your kale, garlic, and lemon zest. Sauté until the greens start wilting
5. Add the rest of the stuffing ingredients and mix well to combine
6. Divide the mix among the fillets, around 2 tablespoons per fillet
7. Cover the top of each fillet with the mustard, and coat with the panko
8. Arrange in a baking tray lined with parchment paper and roast for around 20 minutes.

Nutritional Values (Per Serving)

- Calories: 274
- Fat: 11.6g
- Saturated Fat: 1.6g
- Trans Fat: 0g

- Carbohydrates: 34.4g
- Fiber: 9.8g
- Sodium: 41mg
- Protein: 10g

Vegetarian Lasagna

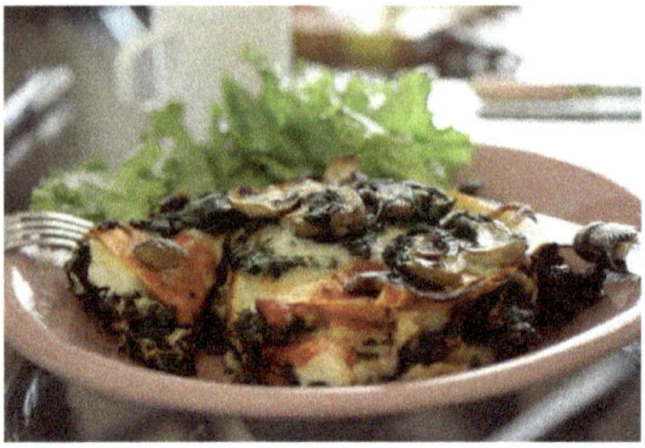

(Prepping Time: 30 minutes | Cooking Time: 60 minutes | For 12 servings)

Ingredients

- 16 whole-wheat lasagna noodles, cooked and drained
- 1 cups onion, minced
- 15oz low fat cottage cheese
- 3 cups canned tomatoes
- 2 zucchinis, diced
- 6 cloves of garlic, minced
- 2 tablespoons margarine 20%
- 2 yellow squash, diced
- 1 12oz jar roasted red peppers, drained and sliced into strips
- 1 cup low-fat parmesan cheese, grated

- 8 ounces low-fat mozzarella cheese, shredded
- basil leaves
- Salt and pepper to taste
- 2 large eggs

How to

1. Preheat oven to 350F
2. Spray a 13" x9" baking dish with cooking spray
3. Drain the cooked noodles and arrange them on the baking dish, covering the bottom
4. Preppingare the vegetables:
5. In a non-stick skillet over medium heat, melt the margarine.
6. Add the onion and sauté until translucent
7. Add the squash, zucchini, and garlic. Add salt to taste and cook for another 8 minutes, stirring occasionally
8. Add the peppers and tomatoes and bring to a gentle simmer.
9. Cook until the liquids have reduced in half, and the sauce begins to thicken (about 5 minutes).
10. Add the basil and season to taste.
11. Pour 1/3 of the vegetable mix over the arranged noodles in the baking dish, forming another layer.
12. Arrange another layer of noodles over the vegetables.
13. In a bowl, mix half a teaspoon of salt, the cottage cheese, and eggs, then pour half of it over the layered noodles.
14. Sprinkle 1/3 of the mozzarella and 1/3 of the parmesan over the cottage cheese mix.
15. Form another layer of vegetables using another 1/3.
16. Repeat until you are out of vegetable and cottage cheese mix.
17. Finish with another layer of noodles, topping with the remaining mixture of parmesan and mozzarella.
18. Cover dish with tinfoil and bake for 20 minutes.
19. Remove tinfoil, then bake for an additional 10 until the cheese browns

20. Let it rest for 5 minutes before serving.

Nutritional Values (Per Serving)

- Calories: 382
- Fat: 6.9g
- Saturated Fat: 1.9g
- Trans Fat: 0.1g
- Carbohydrates: 53.1g
- Fiber: 9.5g
- Sodium: 528mg
- Protein: 24.5g

Shrimp and Cilantro Meal

(Prepping time: 10 minutes | Cooking time: 5 minutes | For 4 servings)

Ingredients

- 1 ¾ pounds shrimp, peeled and deveined
- 2 tablespoons fresh lime juice
- ½ teaspoon ground cumin
- ¼ teaspoon cloves, minced
- 1 tablespoon olive oil
- 1 ¼ cups cilantro, freshly chopped
- 1 teaspoon lime zest
- ½ teaspoon salt
- ¼ teaspoon pepper

How To

1. Take a large-sized bowl and add shrimp, cumin, garlic, lime juice, and
2. ginger. Toss well.
3. Add oil to a large nonstick skillet, and allow it to heat up over medium-
4. high heat.
5. Add shrimp mix and sauté for 4 minutes.
6. Remove from the heat and add cilantro, lime zest, salt, and pepper.
7. Mix well and serve hot!

Nutritional Values (Per Serving)

- Calories: 177
- Fat: 6g
- Carbohydrates: 3g
- Protein: 27g
- Saturated Fat: 2g
- Sodium: 456 mg
- Fiber: 1g

Awesome Prawn Salsa

(Prepping time: 10 minutes | Cooking time: 5 minutes | For 2 servings)

Ingredients

- 2 bananas, sliced and peeled

- 2 cucumbers, peeled, seeded, and diced
- ½ cup fresh mint leaves
- ½ cup fresh cilantro leaves
- 1 teaspoon fresh ginger root
- 1 fresh red chile pepper, sliced
- ¼ cup lime juice
- 1 tablespoon fish sauce
- 1 tablespoon brown sugar
- 1 and ½ pounds peeled and deveined tiger prawns

How To

1. Take a large-sized bowl and add bananas, cucumber, cilantro, ginger, red chile pepper, and mix everything well
2. The above mix is your Salsa
3. Take a small-sized bowl and add lime juice, brown sugar, fish sauce, sugar, and blend
4. Add salsa mix to the fish sauce mixture and stir
5. Take a large saucepan and add salted water
6. Bring the water to a boil
7. Add prawns into the water and cook for 3 minutes
8. Serve the cooked prawn with banana salsa
9. Enjoy!

Nutritional Values (Per Serving)

- Calories: 280
- Fat: 2 g
- Saturated Fat: 0.5 g
- Carbohydrates: 25 g
- Fiber: 1 g
- Sodium: 141 mg
- Protein: 36 g

Perfect Potato Soup

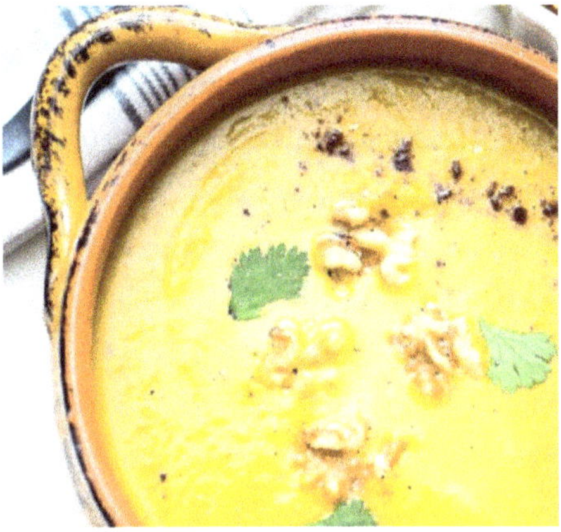

(Prepping time: 10 minutes | Cooking time: 28 minutes | For 4 servings)

Ingredients

- 2 tablespoons extra virgin olive oil
- 1 large onion, chopped
- 2 cloves garlic, crushed
- 1 pound sweet potato, peeled and cut into medium pieces
- ½ teaspoon ground cumin
- ¼ teaspoon ground chili
- ½ teaspoon ground coriander
- ¼ teaspoon ground cinnamon
- ¼ teaspoon salt
- 2 cups chicken stock
- Low fat crème fraiche
- Freshly chopped parsley (as a garnish)
- Coriander as needed

How To

1. Place a large pan over medium-high heat.
2. Add olive oil and heat it up.
3. Add onions and sauté them until they are slightly browned.
4. Turn down the heat to medium, add garlic, and keep cooking for 2-3
5. minutes more.
6. Add sweet potato and sauté for 3-4 minutes.
7. Add the remaining spices.
8. Cook for 2 minutes.
9. Pour stock and turn the heat up.
10. Bring the mixture to a boil and give it a stir.
11. Cover, lower heat, and bring it to a slow simmer.
12. Cook for 20 minutes until the potatoes are tender.
13. Remove the pan from the heat.
14. Take an immersion blender and puree the whole mixture.
15. Add a bit of water if the soup is too thick.
16. Check the soup for seasoning.
17. Ladle the soup into your serving bowls.
18. Give a swirl of crème fraiche.
19. Sprinkle some chopped-up parsley.
20. Enjoy!

Nutritional Values (Per Serving)

- Calories: 324
- Fat: 7g
- Carbohydrates: 25g
- Protein: 12g
- Saturated Fat: 3g
- Sodium: 233 mg
- Fiber: 2g

Heirloom Carrots

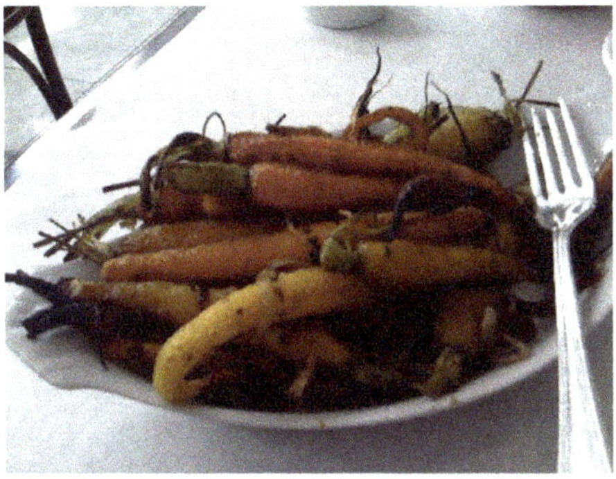

(Prepping time: 10 minutes | Cooking time: 45 minutes | For 4 servings)

Ingredients

- 1 bunch of fine heirloom carrots
- 1 tablespoon fresh thyme leaves
- ½ tablespoon coconut oil
- 1 tablespoon date paste
- 1/8 cup fresh-squeezed orange juice
- 1/8 teaspoon sea salt
- Salt as needed

How To

1. Preheat your Oven to 350 degrees Fahrenheit.
2. Wash the carrots and discard the green pieces.
3. Take a small-sized bowl and add coconut oil, orange juice, date paste, and
4. salt.
5. Place the carrots on a large-sized baking sheet and pour the dressing over
6. them.

7. Sprinkle thyme on top.
8. Roast for 45 minutes.
9. Season with salt, and enjoy!

Nutritional Values (Per Serving)

- Calories: 70
- Fat: 3g
- Carbohydrates: 11g
- Protein: 1g
- Saturated Fat: 1g
- Sodium: 150 mg
- Fiber: 5g

Superb Roasted Cauliflower Fattoush

(Prepping time: 10 minutes | Cooking time: 60 minutes | For 4 servings)

Ingredients

- 3 pounds raw cauliflower, broken up into small florets
- 1 medium red onion, cut up into thin slices
- 2 individual Lebanese wholemeal bread
- 1 cups canned chickpeas, rinsed and drained
- 2 medium tomatoes, coarsely chopped
- 1 cup fresh flat-leaf parsley
- ½ cup no-fat Greek-Style natural yogurt
- 1 teaspoon ground sumac
- 1 tablespoon Dukkah

- 1 tablespoon walnuts
- Cooking spray

How To

1. Preheat your Oven to 390 degrees Fahrenheit.
2. Take a baking tray and line it up with baking paper.
3. Add cauliflower and onion to the tray.
4. Lightly spray with cooking spray.
5. Bake for 45 minutes until tender and golden.
6. While they are being roasted, place the bread on the rack of the Oven and
7. bake for 8 minutes until golden and crisp.
8. Set the bread aside and allow them to cool.
9. Break the bread into small pieces.
10. Place the cauliflower, bread pieces, onion, chickpeas, parsley, and
11. tomatoes in a large bowl.
12. Take a small bowl and add yogurt, sumac, and ¼ cup of water.
13. Season with salt and pepper. Whisk well.
14. Drizzle over salad and toss well.
15. Serve with a sprinkle of walnuts and Dukkah.

Nutritional Values (Per Serving)

- Calories: 240
- Fat: 11g
- Carbohydrates: 31g
- Protein: 9g
- Saturated Fat: 2g
- Sodium: 230 mg
- Fiber: 2g

Exquisite Chicken Taco Bowl

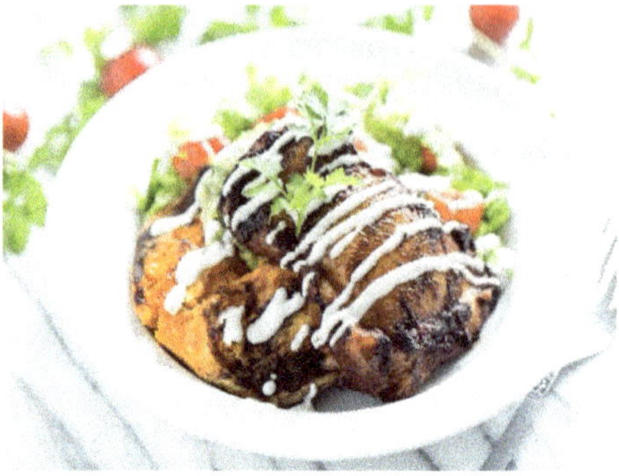

(Prepping time: 10 minutes | Cooking time: 35 minutes | For 4 servings)

Ingredients

- 2 cups chicken, shredded
- 1 onion, diced
- 1 bell pepper, diced
- 1 poblano pepper, diced
- 2 tomatoes, chopped
- 1 tablespoon garlic, minced
- 6 cups fat-free chicken broth
- 1 cup tomato sauce
- 1 ½ cups kidney beans
- 2 tablespoons taco seasoning
- 1 tablespoon olive oil
- Shredded cheese, crushed tortilla chips, or sour cream for serving

How To

1. In a large-sized stockpot, add onion, poblano pepper, bell pepper, and tomato. Sauté over medium-high heat for 5 minutes.
2. Add chicken, broth, tomato sauce, beans, and seasoning.

3. Lower the heat to medium and cook for 30 minutes. Serve with sour cream and cheese, and enjoy!

Nutritional Values (Per Serving)

- Calories: 209
- Fat: 9g
- Carbohydrates: 27g
- Saturated Fat: 3g
- Sodium: 123 mg
- Fiber: 2g

Delish-Chicken Fried Rice

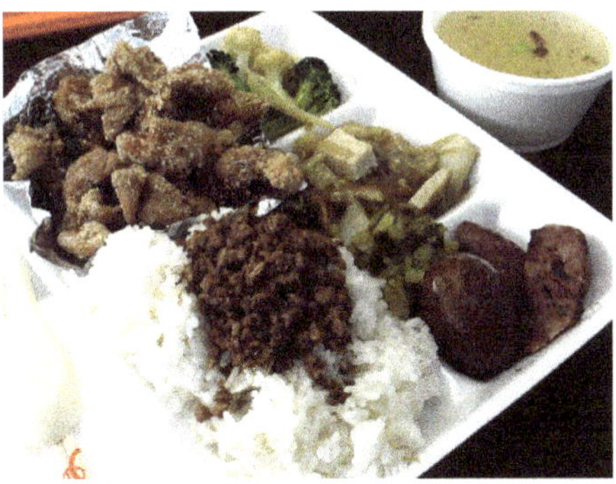

(Prepping time: 10 minutes | Cooking time: 12 minutes | For 4 servings)

Ingredients

- 1 teaspoon olive oil
- 4 large egg whites
- 1 onion, chopped
- 2 garlic cloves, minced
- 12 ounces skinless chicken breasts, boneless, cut into ½ inch cubes

- ½ cup carrots, chopped
- ½ cup of frozen green peas
- 2 cups long-grain brown rice, cooked
- 3 tablespoons soy sauce, low sodium

How To

1. Coat skillet with oil, place it over medium-high heat
2. Add egg whites and cook until scrambled
3. Sauté onion, garlic and chicken breasts for 6 minutes
4. Add carrots, peas and keep cooking for 3 minutes
5. Stir in rice, season with soy sauce
6. Add cooked egg whites, stir for 3 minutes
7. Enjoy!

Nutritional Values (Per Serving)

- Calories: 330
- Fat: 11g
- Carbohydrates: 20g
- Protein: 23g
- Saturated Fat: 3g
- Sodium: 1005mg
- Fiber: 1g

Enticing Mango Chicken

(Prepping time: 10 minutes | Cooking time: 10 minutes | For 4 servings)

Ingredients

- 2 medium mangoes, peeled and sliced
- 10 ounces of coconut milk
- 4 teaspoons olive oil

- 4 teaspoons curry paste
- 14 ounces chicken breasts, skinless and boneless, cut into cubes
- 4 medium shallots
- 1 large English cucumber, seeded and sliced

How To

1. Slice half of the mangoes and add the halves to a bowl
2. Add mangoes and coconut milk to a blender and blend until you have a smooth puree
3. Keep the mixture on the side
4. Take a large-sized pot and place it over medium heat, add oil and allow the oil to heat up
5. Add curry paste and cook for 1 minute until you have a nice fragrance, add shallots and chicken to the pot, and cook for 5 minutes
6. Pour mango puree into the mix and allow it to heat up
7. Serve the cooked chicken with mango puree and cucumbers
8. Enjoy!

Nutritional Values (Per Serving)

- Calories: 400
- Fat: 20 g
- Saturated Fat: 5 g
- Carbohydrates: 31 g
- Fiber: 8 g
- Sodium: 1235 mg
- Protein: 26 g

Onion Dressed Pork Cutlets

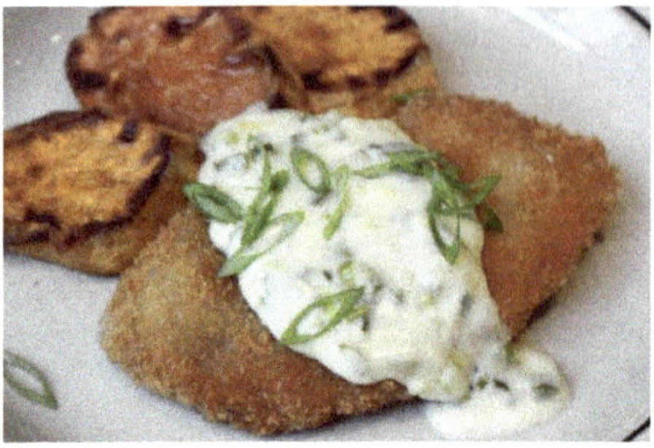

(Prepping time: 10 minutes | Cooking time: 10 minutes | For 4 servings)

Ingredients

- 1 tablespoon olive oil
- 2 pork cutlets
- 1 bell pepper, deveined and sliced
- 1 Spanish onion, chopped
- 2 garlic cloves, minced
- ½ teaspoon hot sauce
- ½ teaspoon mustard
- ½ teaspoon paprika
- Salt and pepper to taste

How To

1. Take a large saucepan, add olive oil and place it over medium-high heat
2. Let it heat up, add pork cutlets and fry for 3-4 minutes until golden and crispy on both sides
3. Lower temperature to medium and add bell pepper, Spanish onion, garlic, hot sauce, mustard and cook for 3 minutes until veggies are tender
4. Sprinkle paprika, salt, pepper and serve
5. Enjoy!

Nutritional Values (Per Serving)

- Calories: 24
- Fat: 3 g
- Saturated Fat: 1 g
- Carbohydrates: 2 g
- Fiber: 0.8 g
- Sodium: 219 mg
- Protein: 40 g

Sushi Bowl

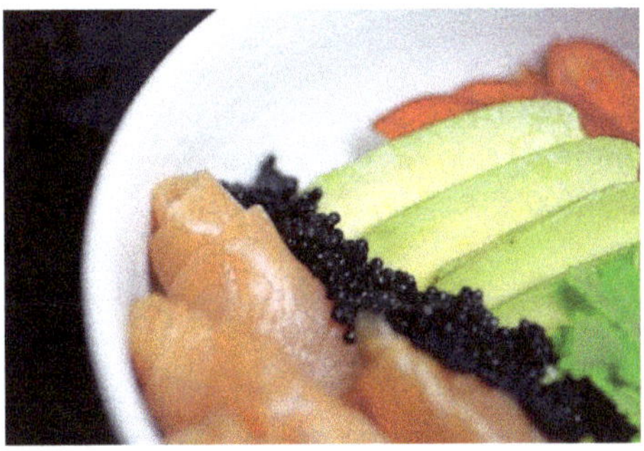

(Prepping Time: 10 minutes | Cooking Time: 5 minutes | For 6 Servings)

Ingredients

- 3 cup(s)s brown rice, cooked (steamed)
- 18 oz shrimp, cleaned and cooked
- 1 1/2 cucumber, thinly sliced
- 1 1/2 avocado, peeled, pitted, and diced
- 1 1/2 cup(s) carrots, carrots
- 4 1/2 tablespoon(s) pickled ginger, thinly chopped
- 6 tablespoon(s) sesame-ginger dressing

How To

1. Divide the rice among 6 bowls.
2. Top with the shrimp, the avocado, the cucumber, the carrot, and the ginger.
3. Drizzle with the sesame ginger dressing over each bowl.
4. If you want you can top with nori before serving (calories and points not included).

Nutritional Values (Per Serving)

- Calories: 339
- Fat: 14.6g
- Saturated Fat: 1.9g
- Trans Fat: 0.1g
- Carbohydrates: 32.7g
- Fiber: 6g
- Sodium: 250mg
- Protein: 21.3g

Roasted Cauliflower

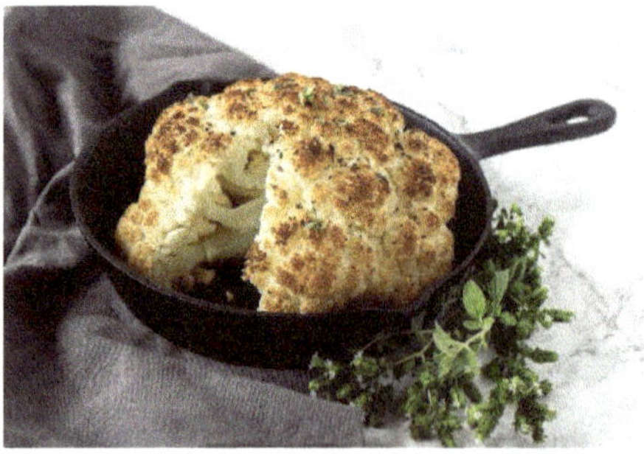

(Prepping Time: 5 minutes | Cooking Time: 20 mins | For 12 Servings)

Ingredients

- 12 cup(s)s cauliflower florets, chopped
- 3 tablespoon(s) Soy sauce
- 3/4 tablespoon(s) canola oil
- 1 teaspoon(s) black pepper
- 1 1/2 teaspoon(s) fructose

How To

1. Preheat your oven to 450F with the rack in the middle of the oven.
2. In a bowl, mix the soy sauce, the oil, the pepper, and the fructose.
3. Add the cauliflower and set aside for 20 minutes.
4. Arrange on a baking sheet lined with parchment paper.
5. Roast for 20 minutes until lightly charred.
6. Serve hot.

Nutritional Values (Per Serving)

- Calories: 40
- Fat: 1.2g
- Saturated Fat: 0.2g
- Trans Fat: 0g
- Carbohydrates: 6g
- Fiber: 2g
- Sodium: 283mg
- Protein: 3g

Strawberry Sorbet

(Prepping Time: 5 minutes+freezing overnight | Cooking Time: 20 minutes | For 8 Servings)

Ingredients

- 8 cup(s)s ripe strawberries, sliced and frozen
- 4 tablespoon(s) Powdered Stevia or another sweetener

How To

1. Peel and slice strawberries in small pieces and freeze overnight
2. Add all of your ingredients in a high-speed blender and pulse for about 6 minutes, stopping every couple of minutes to scrape the sides of the blender.
3. Pulse until the consistency resembles soft-serve.
4. Taste and add more sweetener if you want.
5. Divide among bowls.
6. Freeze for a minimum of 15 minutes before serving.

Nutritional Values (Per Serving)

- Calories: 46
- Fat: 0.4g
- Saturated Fat: 0g
- Trans Fat: 0g
- Carbohydrates: 12g
- Fiber: 3g
- Sodium: 1mg
- Protein: 1g

Citrus carrots

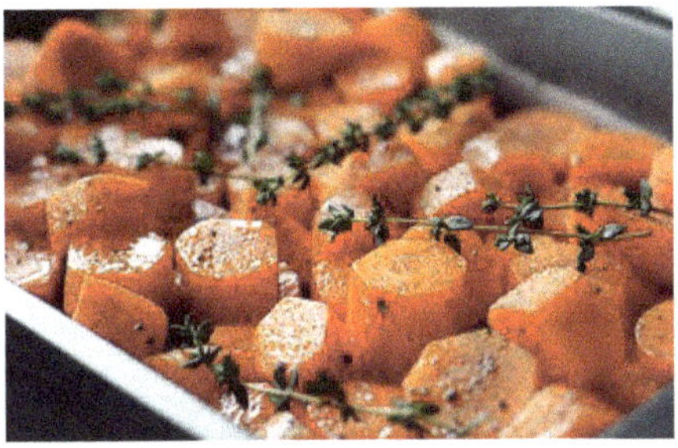

(Prepping Time: 10 min | Cooking Time: 5 min | For 2 Servings)

Ingredients

- 1 ½ cups grated carrot
- 1 teaspoon fresh ginger, minced
- 4 tablespoons fresh orange juice
- 1 teaspoon olive oil
- Salt and black pepper, to taste

How To

1. In a large non-stick pan, add oil, carrot, and ginger over medium-high heat. Stir well.
2. Cook for about 2 minutes and low down the flame.
3. Now, add in orange juice, black pepper and salt and simmer for about 3 minutes.
4. Take out and serve.

Nutritional Values (Per Serving)

- Calories: 71
- Fat: 2.4g
- Saturated Fat: 0.4g
- Trans Fat: 1g
- Carbohydrates: 12g

- Fiber: 2.2g
- Sodium: 135mg
- Protein: 1g

Vegetable Broth with Cabbage

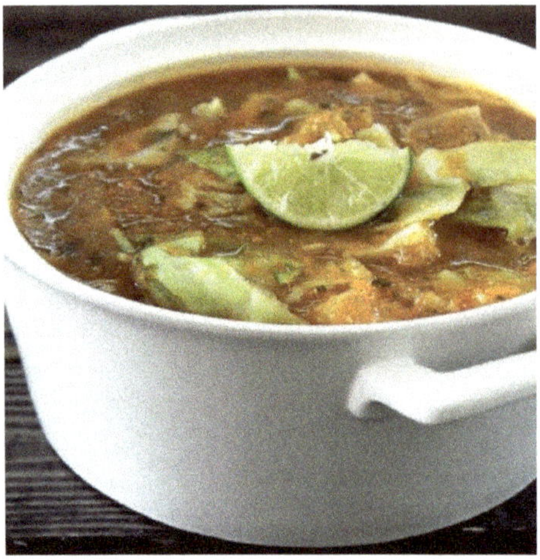

(Prepping Time: 5 min | Cooking Time: 25 min | For 4 Servings)

Ingredients

- 1 cup vegetable broth
- 3 cups green cabbage, chopped
- 1 onion, thinly sliced
- 1 ½ teaspoons extra-virgin olive oil
- Salt and pepper, to taste

How To

1. In a large non-stick skillet, add oil and olive oil over high heat and sauté for about 2 minutes.
2. Now, add cabbage and sauté for about 3 minutes.

3. Add in salt, pepper and broth and reduce the heat to low.
4. Cook for about 20 minutes and take out.
5. Serve hot.

Nutritional Values (Per Serving)

- Calories: 49
- Fat: 2.2g
- Saturated Fat: 0.4g
- Trans Fat: 1.7g
- Carbohydrates: 5.9g
- Fiber: 1.9g
- Sodium: 240mg
- Protein: 2.2g

Baked Chicken Parmesan

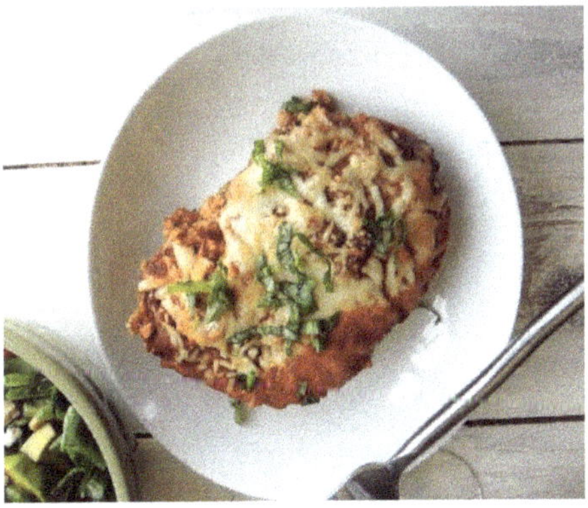

(Prepping Time: 20 min | Cooking Time: 18 min | For 8 Servings)

Ingredients

- 8 (1/2 pound each) boneless and skinless chicken breasts
- 4 tablespoons grated parmesan cheese

- 1 teaspoon salt
- 1 cup reduced-fat mozzarella cheese, shredded
- 4 tablespoons reduced-fat mayonnaise
- 16 basil leaves
- 1 cup panko bread crumbs
- 2 tablespoons olive oil
- 2 large tomatoes cut into 16 slices

How To

1. Preheat the baking oven to 425 degrees F and cover the baking sheet with a non-stick cooking spray.
2. Meanwhile, cover the chicken breasts with salt and mayonnaise.
3. Now, place them (one at a time) in a zipper plastic bag containing the crumbs and shake properly.
4. After that, place them on the baking sheet and top with tomato slices and oil.
5. Put basil leaves on tomato slices and sprinkle mozzarella cheese on them.
6. Bake for about 15-18 minutes until the cheese is melted and becomes light golden.
7. Take out and sprinkle with parmesan cheese.
8. Serve and enjoy!

Nutritional Values (Per Serving)

- Calories: 424
- Fat: 14.4g
- Saturated Fat: 3.6g
- Trans Fat: 5g
- Carbohydrates: 13.3g
- Fiber: 1.2g
- Sodium: 720mg
- Protein: 60.4g

Corn and Tomato Salad

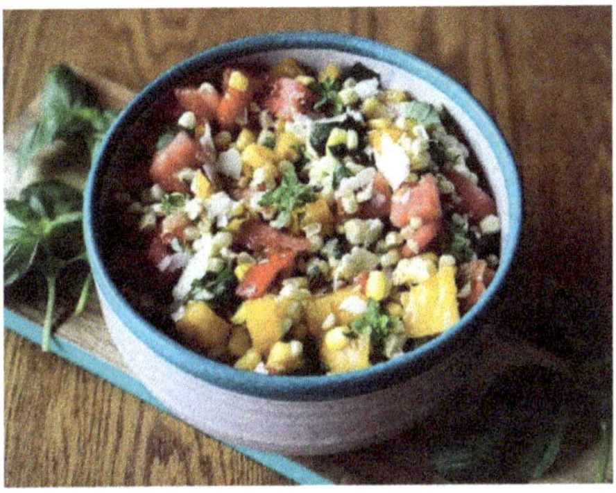

(Prepping Time: 5 min | Cooking Time: 0 min | For 4 Servings)

Ingredients

- 2 tablespoons extra-virgin olive oil
- 2 cups corn kernels
- 3 tablespoons minced shallots
- 3 cups cherry tomatoes, halved
- 1 tablespoon lemon juice
- 2 tablespoons chopped parsley
- ½ teaspoon black pepper
- Salt, to taste

How To

1. In a bowl, add olive oil, tomatoes, shallots, and corn. Mix properly.
2. Now, add in salt, pepper, and lemon juice. Toss well.
3. Top with chopped parsley and serve.

Nutritional Values (Per Serving)

- Calories: 158
- Fat: 8.2g
- Saturated Fat: 1.2g
- Trans Fat: 4.8g
- Carbohydrates: 21.4g
- Fiber: 3.9g
- Sodium: 60mg
- Protein: 4g

Vegetarian Lo Mein

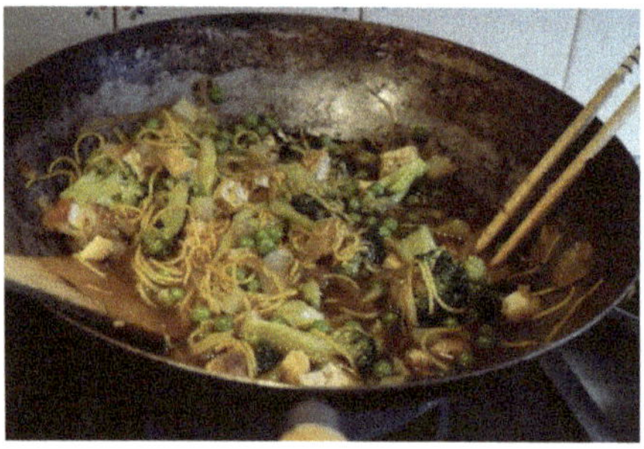

(Prepping Time: 10 minutes | Cooking Time: 15 minutes | For 4 Servings)

Ingredients

- 8oz lo mein, cooked and drained
- 2 cups shiitake mushrooms, sliced
- 3 cloves of garlic, minced
- 3 cups spinach
- 1/2 cup snow peas
- 1 red bell peppers, julienned
- 1 tablespoon margarine 20% fat
- 1 zucchini, julienned

- 1 carrot, julienned
- *For the sauce:*
- 2 tablespoon soy sauce reduced sodium
- 2 teaspoons Splenda
- 1 teaspoon canola oil
- 1/2 teaspoon ginger
- 1/2 teaspoon chili sauce

How To

1. In a bowl, whisk the soy sauce, oil, Splenda, chili sauce, and ginger. Set aside.
2. Set a wok over high heat and add the margarine to heat.
3. Add the vegetables, apart from the peas and the spinach.
4. Cook, stirring often until the vegetables soften, about 4 minutes.
5. Add the peas and spinach. Cook for 3 more minutes, until the spinach wilts
6. Add the sauce mixture and the noodles. Toss gently to combine
7. Serve immediately

Nutritional Values (Per Serving)

- Calories: 175
- Fat: 2.5g
- Saturated Fat: 0.3g
- Trans Fat: 0g
- Carbohydrates: 35.8g
- Fiber: 4.5g
- Sodium: 513mg
- Protein: 5.1g

Thai salad with nut and curry dressing

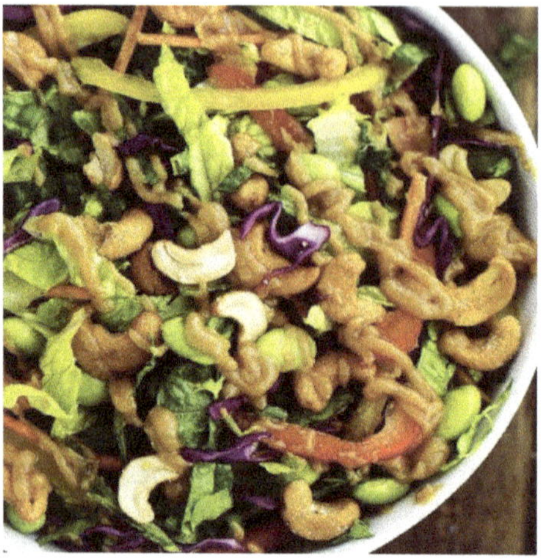

(Prepping Time: 10 minutes | Cooking Time: 60 minutes | For 16 Servings)

Ingredients

For the dressing:

- 4 tablespoons curry powder
- 6 tablespoons peanut butter powder
- 6 tablespoons water
- 2 teaspoon salt
- 4 cups unsweetened coconut milk
- *For the Salad:*
- 4 mangoes, chopped
- ¾ cup freshly squeezed lime juice
- 11oz (2 2/3 cups) pepitas
- 1 cup lettuce, shredded
- 2 avocados, in small dice
- 16 green onion stalks, roughly chopped
- 2 red peppers, in strips
- 1 cup kale, shredded

- 1 cup spinach, shredded
- 1 cup cabbage, shredded

How To

For the Dressing:

1. Add all the ingredients to a food processor and blend until smooth.
2. Set aside in the fridge for around 2 hours or until it has thickened
3. For the Salad:
4. Add the ingredients into a salad bowl toss.
5. Drizzle with the dressing before serving

Nutritional Values (Per Serving)

- Calories: 279
- Fat: 17.6g
- Saturated Fat: 3.5g
- Trans Fat: 0.5g
- Carbohydrates: 25.8g
- Fiber: 6.3g
- Sodium: 347mg
- Protein: 11.1g

Gazpacho

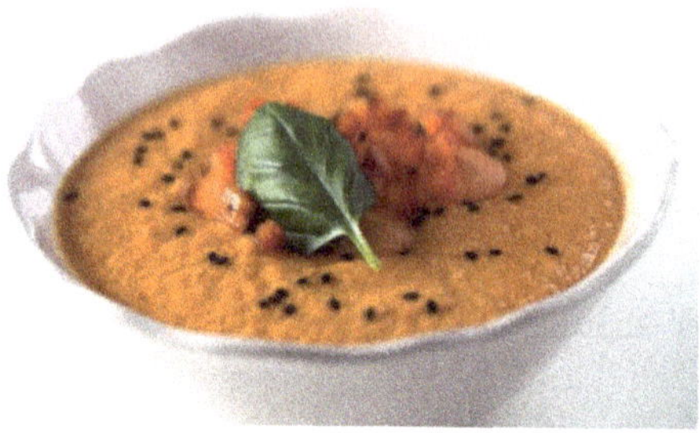

(Prepping Time: 15 minutes | Cooking Time: 30 minutes + an additional hour to chill | For 4 Servings)

Ingredients

- 4 cups canned tomatoes, chunkily chopped
- 1 avocado, peeled, pitted, and diced
- 2 cups vegetable stock
- 3 green onions, finely chopped
- 3 leeks, finely chopped
- 2 bay leaves
- 4 cloves of garlic, minced
- 1 cup of water
- 1/4 teaspoon salt

How To

1. Add all the ingredients apart from the stock and avocados in a pot and simmer for 30 minutes.
2. Add the stock and simmer for another 15 minutes.
3. Use a mesh sieve lined with a cotton fabric to strain the soup.
4. Chill for at least an hour.
5. Divide into bowls and add the avocados

Nutritional Values (Per Serving)

- Calories: 164
- Fat: 10g
- Saturated Fat: 2.2g
- Trans Fat: 0g
- Carbohydrates: 14.1g
- Fiber: 6.3g
- Sodium: 545mg
- Protein: 5.6g

Parmesan-crust Tilapia

(Prepping Time: 10 minutes | Cooking Time: 12 minutes | For 8 Servings)

Ingredients

- 2lb tilapia fillets
- 1/2 cup fat-free Parmesan cheese
- 4 tablespoons margarine 20% fat, softened
- 4 tablespoons fat-free mayonnaise
- 2 tablespoon fresh lemon juice
- 1/4 teaspoon basil
- 1/4 teaspoon black pepper
- 1/4 teaspoon onion powder
- 1/8 teaspoon garlic powder
- 1/4 teaspoon celery seeds

How To

1. Preheat your broiler.
2. Line a broiling pan with parchment paper.

3. Mix all of the ingredients apart from the fish in a bowl. Stir until evenly combined.
4. Place the fillets on the pan.
5. Broil only a few inches away from the broiler for about 3 minutes on each side.
6. Take fillets out from oven and cover with the mixture on the top side.
7. Broil for another couple of minutes until the cheese mix has browned.
8. Serve immediately.

Nutritional Values (Per Serving)

- Calories: 114
- Fat: 2.8g
- Saturated Fat: 0.7g
- Trans Fat: 0g
- Carbohydrates: 1.1g
- Fiber: 0.2g
- Sodium: 164mg
- Protein: 21.2g

Juicy Teriyaki Salmon

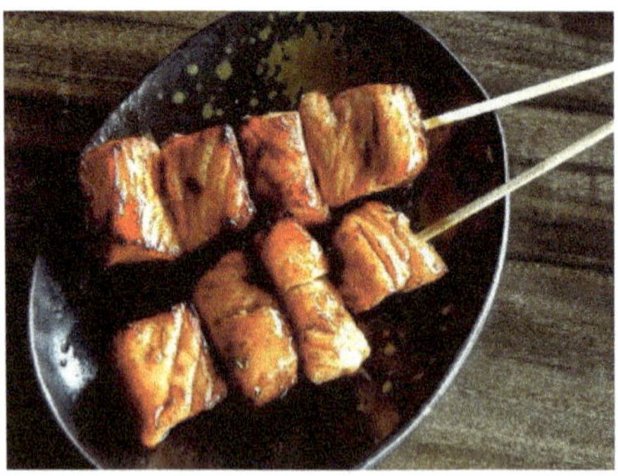

(Prepping time: 10 minutes | Cooking time: 20 minutes | For 4 servings)

Ingredients

- ¼ cup dry sherry
- ¼ cup low-sodium soy sauce
- 1 tablespoon brown sugar
- 1 tablespoon rice wine vinegar
- 1 teaspoon garlic powder
- ½ teaspoon ginger
- 1/8 teaspoon ground black pepper
- 16 ounces salmon fillet skinless, about 1 inch thick
- Cooking spray

How To

1. Take a shallow dish and add sherry, brown sugar, garlic powder, soy
2. sauce, vinegar, ginger, and pepper. Mix well.
3. Add the fish.
4. Allow the fish to marinate for 30 minutes.
5. Coat your grill rack with cooking spray and set it to medium-hot coals
6. allowing the temperature to reach 350-400 degrees Fahrenheit.
7. Remove the fish from the marinade and place it on the grill, cook for 6
8. minutes per side, reserving the marinade for later use.
9. Transfer the grilled fish to a serving platter and keep it warm by placing it
10. under an aluminum tent.
11. Transfer the reserved marinade to a small saucepan and boil for 5
12. minutes until it has a syrup-like texture.
13. Spoon the mix over the fish and serve!

Nutritional Values (Per Serving)

- Calories: 182
- Fat: 5g
- Carbohydrates: 6g
- Protein: 24g
- Saturated Fat: 2g
- Sodium: 256 mg
- Fiber: 1g

The Mediterranean Fish Delight

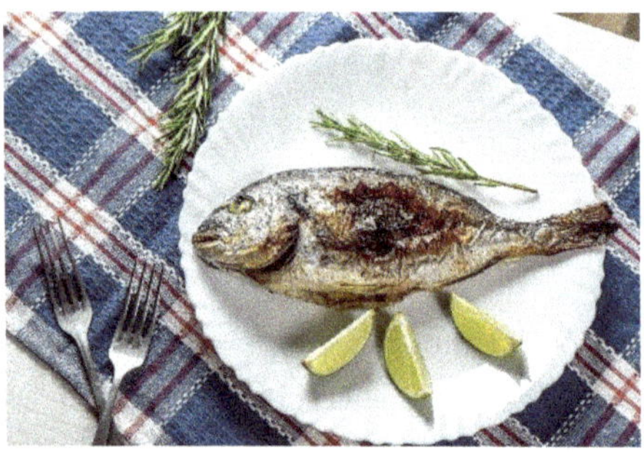

(Prepping time: 10 minutes | Cooking time: 25 minutes | For 4 servings)

Ingredients

- 2 tablespoons olive oil
- 4 pieces (6 ounces each) fish fillets
- 1 large tomato, chopped
- ¼ cup pitted olives, low sodium
- 2 tablespoons capers
- 1 tablespoon lemon juice
- Salt and pepper to taste

How To

1. Preheat your Oven to 350 degrees F
2. Place olive oil in the middle of a large aluminum foil, put fish in the middle, and top with tomato, onion, olives, and capers
3. Season well with lemon juice, salt, and pepper
4. Fold in aluminum foil and seal edges well
5. Transfer to baking pan and bake for 25 minutes
6. Serve and enjoy!

Nutritional Values (Per Serving)

- Calories: 210
- Fat: 9g
- Carbohydrates: 13g
- Protein: 27g
- Saturated Fat: 3g
- Sodium: 425 mg
- Fiber: 3g

Turmeric Soup

(Prepping time: 10 minutes | Cooking time: 25 minutes | For 4 Servings)

Ingredients

- 5 teaspoons vegan stock
- 2 ½ cups chopped carrots
- ½ inch nub fresh ginger
- 3 ½ ounces walnuts
- 1 teaspoon turmeric
- ½ teaspoon cumin
- ½ teaspoon cinnamon

- 1 teaspoon garlic powder
- 1 teaspoon lemon juice
- 1 teaspoon chipotle paste

How To

1. Add the listed ingredients to a stockpot.
2. Place it over medium-high heat and bring the mixture to a boil.
3. Once boiling point is reached, immediately lower down the heat to low
4. Simmer on low heat for 25 minutes.
5. Blend the whole mixture using an immersion blender.
6. Enjoy!

Nutritional Values (Per Serving)

- Calories: 208
- Fat: 4g
- Carbohydrates: 35g
- Protein: 10
- Saturated Fat: 2g
- Sodium: 222 mg
- Fiber: 3g

Avocado And Cilantro Delight

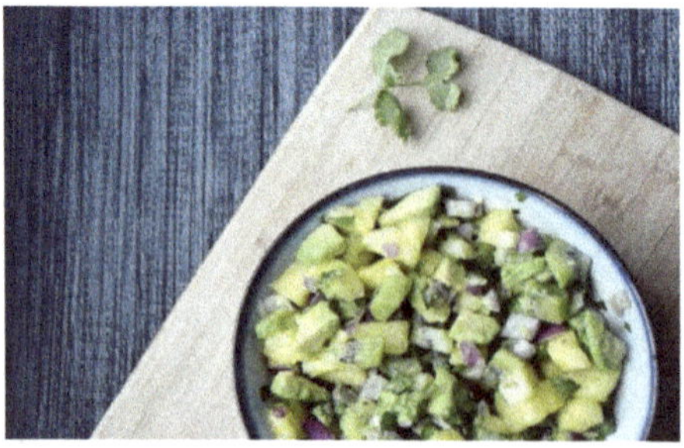

(Prepping time: 10 minutes | Cooking time: 0 minutes | For 4 servings)

Ingredients

- 2 avocados, peeled, pitted, and diced
- 1 sweet onion, chopped
- 1 green bell pepper, chopped
- 1 large ripe tomato, chopped
- ¼ cup fresh cilantro, chopped
- ½ lime, juiced
- Salt and pepper to taste

How To

1. Take a medium-sized bowl and add onion, avocados, tomatoes, bell pepper, lime juice, and cilantro
2. Toss well to coat everything
3. Season with salt and pepper
4. Serve chilled!

Nutritional Values (Per Serving)

- Calories: 126
- Fat: 10 g
- Saturated Fat: 2 g
- Carbohydrates: 10 g
- Fiber: 2 g
- Sodium: 65 mg
- Protein: 2 g

Lovely Orange Chicken

(Prepping time: 10 minutes | Cooking time: 35 minutes | For 4 servings)

Ingredients

- 2 tablespoons orange juice
- 2 tablespoons Dijon mustard
- ¼ teaspoon salt
- ¾ cup whole wheat crackers, crumbled
- 1 tablespoon orange zest, grated
- 1 shallot, finely chopped
- ¼ teaspoon freshly ground black pepper
- 12 ounces chicken thighs, boneless and skinless

How To

1. Preheat your Oven to 350 degrees Fahrenheit.
2. Take a nonstick baking sheet and spray with cooking spray.
3. Take a small bowl and add orange juice, mustard, and salt.
4. Take a sheet of wax paper and add cracker crumbs, shallot, orange zest,
5. and pepper.
6. Brush the chicken with the mustard mixture and dredge them in the
7. crumble.
8. Firmly press the coating to ensure that the chicken thighs are coated well.
9. Transfer chicken to the baking sheet.
10. Bake for 15 minutes, turn over and bake for 15 minutes more.
11. Serve and enjoy!

Nutritional Values (Per Serving)

- Calories: 194
- Fat: 7g
- Carbohydrates: 15g

- Protein: 19g
- Saturated Fat: 2g
- Sodium: 267 mg
- Fiber: 3g

Mexi-Chicken Breast

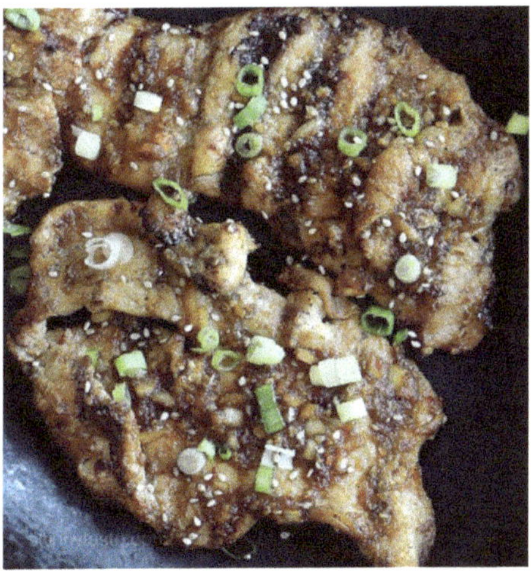

(Prepping time: 10 minutes | Cooking time: 30 minutes | For 4 servings)

Ingredients

- ¼ cup fat-free sour cream
- 1 cup of Salsa
- 4 ounces boneless and skinless chicken breast
- ¼ ounce taco seasoning mix

How To

1. Preheat your Oven to 375 degrees F
2. Transfer chicken breast to a resealable bag
3. Add taco seasoning and shake the bag well until coated
4. Take your casserole dish and grease with cooking spray
5. Add the prepared breast to the casserole
6. Bake for 30 minutes
7. Top with Salsa, and cook for 5 minutes more
8. Top with sour cream
9. Enjoy!

Nutritional Values (Per Serving)

- Calories: 178
- Fat: 3g
- Carbohydrates: 12g
- Protein: 26g
- Saturated Fat: 1g
- Sodium: 304mg
- Fiber: 2g

Southwestern Pork Chops

(Prepping time: 10 minutes | Cooking time: 13 minutes | For 4 servings)

Ingredients

- Vegetable cooking oil spray
- 4 ounces pork loin chop, boneless and trimmed of fat

- 1/3 cup Salsa
- 2 tablespoons fresh lime juice
- ¼ cup fresh cilantro, chopped (optional)

How To

1. Coat a large nonstick skillet with cooking spray.
2. Heat it up until hot over high heat.
3. Press the chops with your palm to flatten them slightly.
4. Add them to the skillet and cook for 1 minute on each side until they are
5. nicely browned.
6. Reduce the heat to medium-low.
7. Combine the Salsa and lime juice.
8. Pour the mix over the chops.
9. Simmer uncovered for about 8 minutes until the chops are perfectly done.
10. If desired, sprinkle some cilantro on top.
11. Serve!

Nutritional Values (Per Serving)

- Calories: 184
- Fat: 8g
- Carbohydrates: 2g
- Protein: 25g
- Saturated Fat: 2g
- Sodium: 369 mg
- Fiber: 2g

Peppered Up Beef Tenderloin

(Prepping time: 10 minutes | Cooking time: 20 minutes | For 4 servings)

Ingredients

- 2 teaspoons sage, chopped
- Salt and pepper
- 2 and1/2 pounds beef tenderloin
- 2 teaspoon thyme, chopped
- 2 garlic cloves, sliced
- 2 teaspoons rosemary, chopped
- 4 teaspoons olive oil

How To

1. Preheat your Oven to 425 degrees F
2. Take a small knife and cut incisions on tenderloin; insert one slice of garlic into the incision
3. Rub meat with oil
4. Take a bowl and add salt, sage, thyme, rosemary, pepper, and mix well
5. Rub spice mix over tenderloin
6. Put rubbed tenderloin into roasting pan and bake for 10 minutes
7. Lower temperature to 350 degrees F and cook for 20 minutes more until an internal thermometer read 145 degrees F
8. Transfer tenderloin to cutting board and let them sit for 15 minutes, slice into 20 pieces, and enjoy!

Nutritional Values (Per Serving)

- Calories: 183

- Fat: 9g
- Carbohydrates: 1g
- Protein: 24g
- Saturated Fat: 3g
- Sodium: 2134mg
- Fiber: 0.1g

Chickpea Burgers

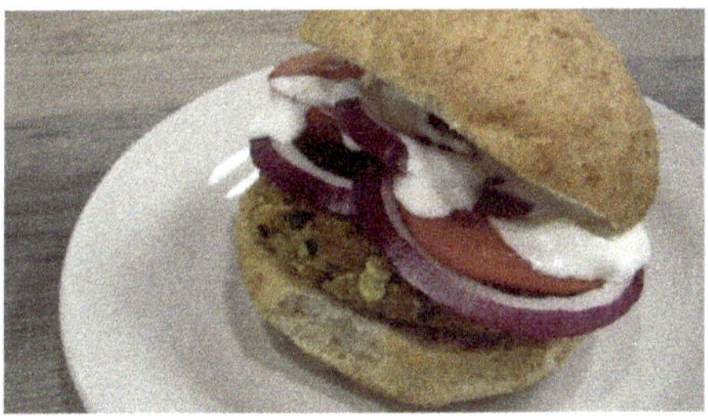

(Prepping Time: 15 minutes | Cooking Time: 100 minutes | For 20 patties)

Ingredients

- 4 1/2 cup(s)s chickpeas, cooked, rinsed and drained
- 3oz shallots, minced
- 6 tablespoon(s) parsley, finely chopped
- 3/4 cup(s) carrots, minced
- 6 tablespoon(s) olive oil
- 3 tablespoon(s) fresh lemon juice
- 1 1/2 tablespoon(s) tomato paste
- 3 teaspoon(s) paprika
- 6 cloves of garlic, minced

- 1 1/2 cup(s) bread crumbs

How To

1. In a large pot add the chickpeas and 6 cup(s)s of water.
2. Bring to a slow boil and allow the chickpeas to simmer until they are soft, around 90 minutes
3. Skip the steps above if you are using canned chickpeas.
4. Drain the chickpeas but save the water and set aside both.
5. Heat the olive oil in a pan, then add the shallots, parsley, carrots, and garlic. M until the parsley starts to wilt
6. Add the lemon juice, tomato paste, paprika, and chickpeas and mash roughly with a fork.
7. Add the chickpea water you saved and keep cooking until all liquids have evaporated.
8. Let cool then add bread crumbs until the mixture becomes pliable.
9. Form the patties then set under a broiler for 7 minutes.

Nutritional Values (Per Serving)

- Calories: 112
- Fat: 5.2g
- Saturated Fat: 0.7g
- Trans Fat: 0g
- Carbohydrates: 13g
- Fiber: 3g
- Sodium: 21mg
- Protein: 4g

Jalapeno Poppers

(Prepping Time: 25 minutes | Cooking Time: 20 minutes | For 6 servings)

Ingredients

- 6 jalapeno peppers
- 3 oz low fat cream cheese, softened
- 1/2 teaspoon(s) garlic powder
- 2 oz low fat sharp cheddar, shredded
- 1 tablespoon(s) chives, finely chopped
- 2 tablespoon(s) bread crumbs
- 1/2 tablespoon(s) 20% fat margarine, melted

How To

1. Preheat your oven to 400F.
2. Wear gloves and slice the jalapenos in half along the length. Scoop out the insides.
3. Put the cream cheese, garlic powder, cheddar cheese, and the chives in a bowl and mix thoroughly.
4. In another bowl, mix the bread crumbs with the margarine.
5. Fill the jalapenos with the cheese mixture.
6. Top with crumbs mixture.
7. Arrange on a baking sheet lined with parchment paper and bake for about 20 minutes, until golden.
8. Allow to cool for at least 5 minutes before serving.

Nutritional Values (Per Serving)

- Calories: 92
- Fat: 3.6g
- Saturated Fat: 1.9g

- Trans Fat: 0g
- Carbohydrates: 10g
- Fiber: 1g
- Sodium: 217 mg
- Protein: 5g

Tuna Crudo

(Prepping Time: 10 mins | Cooking Time: 5 mins | For 8 servings)

Ingredients

- 16 oz tuna, make sure it is even in shape.
- 4 tablespoon(s) lemon juice
- 2 tablespoon(s) canola oil
- 4 teaspoon(s) lemon zest
- 1/2 teaspoon(s) sea salt flakes
- 8 peppermint leaves
- 4 teaspoon(s) microgreens

How To

1. Put the fish in the freezer for 10 minutes to firm it up.
2. Using a sharp knife, slice the fish very thinly
3. Arrange on 8 plates with the slices overlapping slightly.
4. Mix the lemon juice with the canola oil and drizzle over the slices.
5. Sprinkle with the lemon zest
6. Top with the mint leaves and the microgreens
7. Serve immediately.

Nutritional Values (Per Serving)

- Calories: 95
- Fat: 3.8g
- Saturated Fat: 0.4g
- Trans Fat: 0g
- Carbohydrates: 1g
- Fiber: 0g
- Sodium: 171mg
- Protein: 14g

Spinach and Cheese Pasta Bake

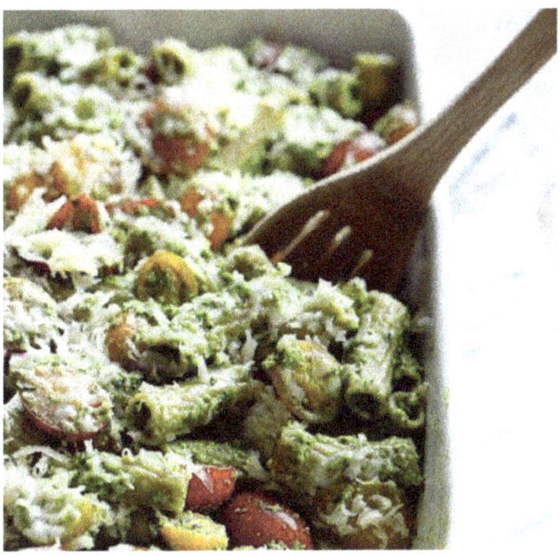

(Prepping Time: 25 minutes | Cooking Time: 25 minutes | For 8 servings)

Ingredients

- 12 oz whole-wheat pasta

- 6 cup(s)s spinach
- 1 medium zucchini, chopped
- 2/3 cup(s) fat free cottage cheese
- 2/3 cup(s) low fat ricotta cheese
- 1 egg white
- 1 teaspoon(s) garlic powder
- 1 Tablespoon(s) Parmesan cheese, shredded
- 1 1/4 cup(s) low-sodium tomato sauce
- 1/3 cup(s) fat free mozzarella cheese, shredded
- salt and pepper to taste

How To

1. Preheat your oven to 350F
2. Cook your pasta according to the box, for 2 minutes less than it requires to be al dente. Strain and set aside.
3. Put the spinach and the zucchini in a microwave-safe bowl. Microwave for 90 seconds on medium-high.
4. In a separate bowl thoroughly mix the garlic powder, the parmesan, and the egg white.
5. Pour the parmesan mixture in the spinach and zucchini, and add the ricotta and cottage cheeses. Mix thoroughly.
6. In a baking pan, pour half of the tomato sauce.
7. Place your half-cooked pasta in the dish and pour the cheese mixture over it. Mix gently.
8. Cover with the remaining tomato sauce.
9. Sprinkle with the mozzarella cheese and bake for 25 minutes until the cheese browns.
    i. Serve hot

Nutritional Values (Per Serving)

- Calories: 293
- Fat: 3.8g

- Saturated Fat: 1.8g
- Trans Fat: 0g
- Carbohydrates: 50g
- Fiber: 6g
- Sodium: 136mg
- Protein: 19g

Spinach Chips

(Prepping Time: 10 min | Cooking Time: 8 min | For 2 servings)

Ingredients

- 1/8 teaspoon olive oil
- 1/8 teaspoon ground cumin
- ¼ teaspoon paprika
- 4 cups fresh spinach leaves
- 1 red chili, chopped
- ½ teaspoon black pepper
- ½ teaspoon salt

How to

1. Line a baking sheet with parchment paper and preheat the baking oven to 325 degrees F.
2. Add oil and spinach leaves in a bowl and mix well until every leave has oil on it.
3. Now, add paprika, ground cumin, chopped red chili, salt, and pepper in that bowl. Stir well.

4. Arrange spinach leaves on the baking sheet and bake for about 8 minutes.
5. Take out and serve.

Nutritional Values (Per Serving)

- Calories: 20
- Fat: 0.6g
- Saturated Fat: 0.1g
- Trans Fat: 0.5g
- Carbohydrates: 2.9g
- Fiber: 1.6g
- Sodium: 630mg
- Protein: 1.9g

Pork and Carrot Stew

(Prepping Time: 10 min | Cooking Time: 8 hours | For 4 servings)

Ingredients

- 1 pound pork meat, trimmed
- 1 cup vegetable broth
- 1 ½ onions sliced
- 3 carrots, peeled and sliced thinly
- ½ teaspoon turmeric
- 1 teaspoon red chili powder
- Salt and pepper, to taste

How to

1. Add all the ingredients in a slow cooker and stir well.
2. Cook for about 8 hours on a low flame.
3. Take out and serve hot.

Nutritional Values (Per Serving)

- Calories: 413
- Fat: 34.8g
- Saturated Fat: 12.4g
- Trans Fat: 11.9g
- Carbohydrates: 8.4g
- Fiber: 1.4g
- Sodium: 1729mg
- Protein: 15.9g

Stir Fried Shrimp

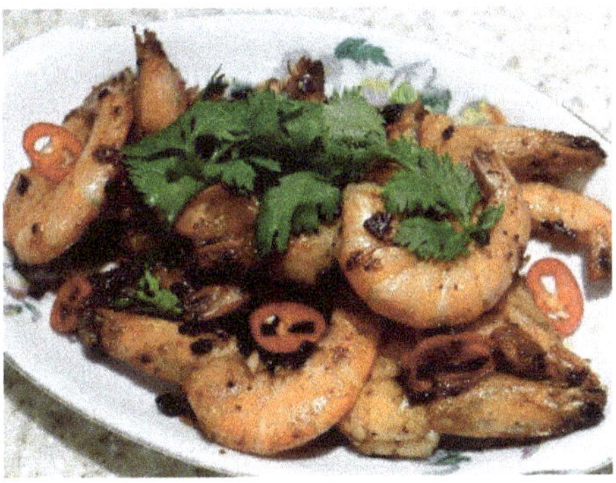

(Prepping Time: 20 min | Cooking Time: 6 min | For 6 servings)

Ingredients

- 2 pounds raw jumbo shrimps, deveined and peeled
- 2 tablespoons olive oil
- 8 garlic cloves, minced
- 8 tablespoons tamari
- Salt and black pepper, to taste

How to

1. Sauté oil and garlic in a large skillet for about 1 minute.
2. Now, add tamari, shrimps, black pepper, and salt. Cook for about 5 minutes.
3. Take out and serve.

Nutritional Values (Per Serving)

- Calories: 168
- Fat: 4.7g
- Saturated Fat: 0.7g
- Trans Fat: 3.2g
- Carbohydrates: 2.7g
- Fiber: 0.3g
- Sodium: 3123mg
- Protein: 29.8g

Parsley Baked Salmon

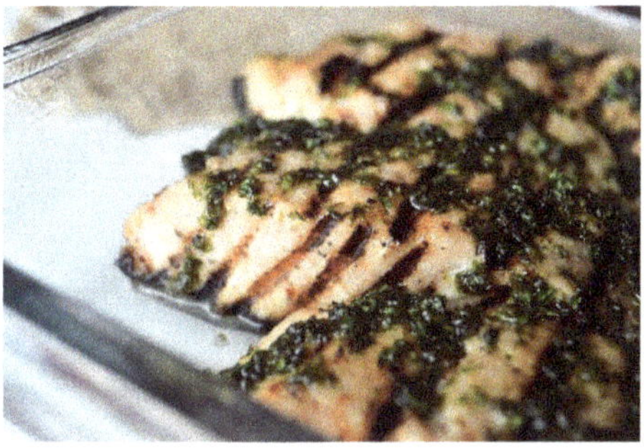

(Prepping Time: 10 min | Cooking Time: 20 min | For 12 servings)

Ingredients

- 4 pounds salmon fillets
- ½ teaspoon ginger powder
- 6 tablespoons fresh parsley, minced
- 3 tablespoons olive oil
- 3 tablespoons lemon juice
- Salt and pepper, to taste

How to

1. Preheat the oven to 400 degrees F.
2. Grease a baking dish and place salmon fillets on it.
3. Drizzle it with olive oil and lemon juice and sprinkle parsley, ginger powder, salt, and black pepper on it.
4. Bake for about 20 minutes and take out.
5. Serve and enjoy!

Nutritional Values (Per Serving)

- Calories: 232

- Fat: 12.9g
- Saturated Fat: 1.9g
- Trans Fat: 5.5g
- Carbohydrates: 0.3g
- Fiber: 0.1g
- Sodium: 69mg
- Protein: 29.4g

Lentil Burgers

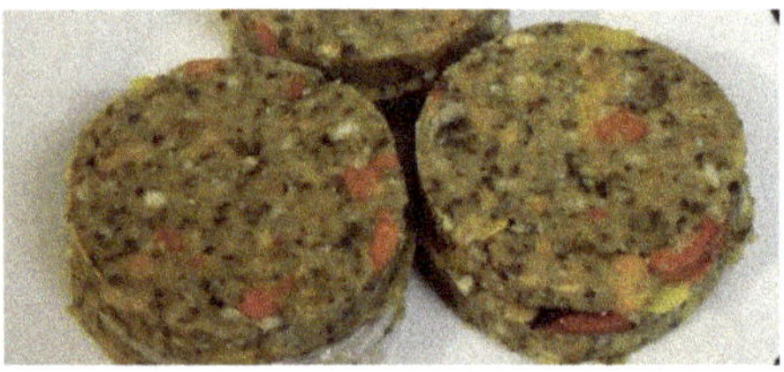

(Prepping Time: 15 minutes | Cooking Time: 90 minutes | For 20 patties)

Ingredients

- 4 1/2 cups lentils, cooked, rinsed, and drained
- 3oz shallots, minced
- 6 tablespoons parsley, finely chopped
- 3/4 cup carrots, finely grated
- 6 tablespoon canola oil
- 3 tablespoon fresh lemon juice
- 1 1/2 tablespoon tomato paste
- 3 teaspoons sweet paprika
- 6 cloves of garlic, minced

- 1 1/2 cup panko

How to

1. In a large pot, add the beans and 6 cups of water, then bring to a slow boil.
2. Let beans simmer until they're soft, around an hour and a half
3. Skip the steps above if using canned.
4. Drain the beans, but save the water and set aside both.
5. In a saucepan, heat the olive oil, then add the shallots, parsley, carrots, and garlic and mix until the parsley begins to wilt
6. Add the lemon juice, tomato paste, paprika, and beans, then mash roughly using a fork or hand blender
7. Add the bean water you have saved and continue cooking until all liquids have evaporated.
8. Let it cool, then add the panko until the mixture becomes pliable.
9. Form the patties, then set under broiler for 5 minutes.

Nutritional Values (Per Serving)

- Calories: 231
- Fat: 5.2g
- Saturated Fat: 0.5g
- Trans Fat: 0g
- Carbohydrates: 33.7g
- Fiber: 13.9g
- Sodium: 68mg
- Protein: 12.6g

Lasagna in a skillet

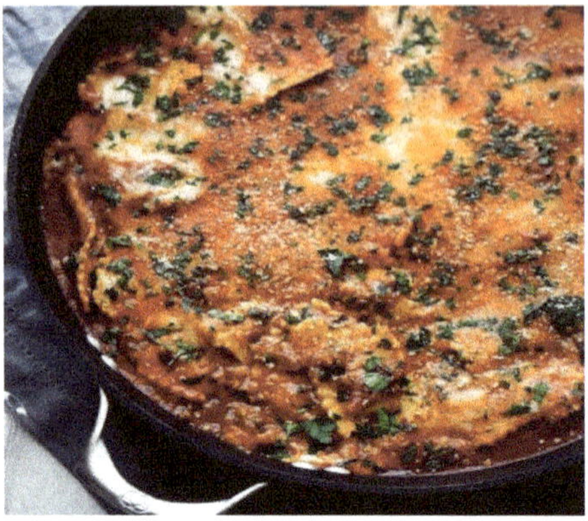

(Prepping Time: 30 minutes | Cooking Time: 30 minutes | For 8 servings)

Ingredients

- 2lb ground turkey
- 2 small onions, chopped
- 6 cloves of garlic, minced
- 2 14oz cans of diced tomatoes, undrained
- 2 1/2 cups water
- 16oz tomato sauce
- 2 tablespoon parsley flakes
- 2 teaspoon basil leaves
- 2 teaspoon oregano
- 2 teaspoon salt
- 5 cups whole wheat lasagna noodles, broken up
- 2 cups fat-free cottage cheese
- 3/4 cup fat-free Parmesan cheese, grated
- 2 eggs

How to

1. Score the eggplants 2-3 times on each side with a knife.
2. Pour 2 cups of water in the Instant Pot® and place the steamer rack trivet in.
3. Place the eggplants on the rack
4. Seal and lock the lid and the vent, select the Manual setting and set it on High pressure for 20 minutes.
5. Turn the vent knob to vent to do a quick release before opening the lid. The eggplants should be completely soft and deflated. Set aside.
6. Set your Instant Pot® on the Sauté setting on High.
7. Add the oil and allow to heat.
8. Add the curry powder, cumin, and turmeric to the inner pot and cook for about half a minute.
9. Add the onions and stir, so they're coated with spices and oil.
10. Cook until the onions are brown and soft, stirring on occasion, around 6 minutes.
11. Add the garlic and ginger and stir. Cook until the garlic softens around a minute.
12. Add tomatoes and cook for about 6 minutes,
13. Chop the eggplant into chunks.
14. Add eggplant and peas to the pot and cook for 3 minutes.
15. Salt and pepper to taste.
16. Serve hot

Nutritional Values (Per Serving)

- Calories: 302
- Fat: 10.3g
- Saturated Fat: 2.1g
- Trans Fat: 0g
- Carbohydrates: 19.5g
- Fiber: 3.5g

- Sodium: 858mg
- Protein: 31.4g

Perfect Oven Baked Tilapia

(Prepping time: 10 minutes | Cooking time: 10 minutes | For 4 servings)

Ingredients

- 1 ½ pound fresh haddock or tilapia fillets
- ¼ cup white cornmeal
- ¼ cup plain bread crumbs
- ½ teaspoon dried dill
- ½ teaspoon salt
- 1/8 teaspoon black pepper
- ½ teaspoon paprika
- 1/3 cup skim milk
- 3 tablespoons butter, melted

How To

1. Preheat your Oven to 450 degrees Fahrenheit.
2. Take a shallow dish and add the listed "Dry" ingredients.
3. Take another dish and add the Milk.
4. Dip the fish into the milk and then dredge in the dry crumb mixture.
5. Place the fish in your pan and evenly coat it with cooking spray.
6. Drizzle melted butter on top.
7. Bake for 10 minutes until the fish is flaky.

8. Serve crispy and enjoy!

Nutritional Values (Per Serving)

- Calories: 196
- Fat: 7g
- Carbohydrates: 8g
- Protein: 20g
- Saturated Fat: 2g
- Sodium: 158 mg
- Fiber: 4g

The Dijon Fish Medley

(Prepping time: 10 minutes | Cooking time: 12 minutes | For 4 servings)

Ingredients

- 1 6-8 ounce fillet of perch, flounder, or sole
- 1 tablespoon Dijon mustard
- 1 ½ teaspoon lemon juice
- 1 teaspoon reduced-sodium Worcestershire sauce
- 2 tablespoons Italian-seasoned bread crumbs
- butter-flavored cooking spray

How To

1. Preheat your Oven to 450 degrees Fahrenheit.
2. Take an 11 x 7-inch baking dish and arrange your fish fillet
3. In a small bowl, mix together the lemon juice, mustard, and

4. Worcestershire sauce.
5. Pour the mixture over the fillet.
6. Sprinkle breadcrumbs on top.
7. Bake for 12 minutes until the fish flakes.
8. Cut the fillet in half and serve.
9. Enjoy!

Nutritional Values (Per Serving)

- Calories: 125
- Fat: 2g
- Carbohydrates: 6g
- Protein: 21g
- Saturated Fat: 0.5g
- Sodium: 257 mg
- Fiber: 1g

Zucchini Wrapped Fish

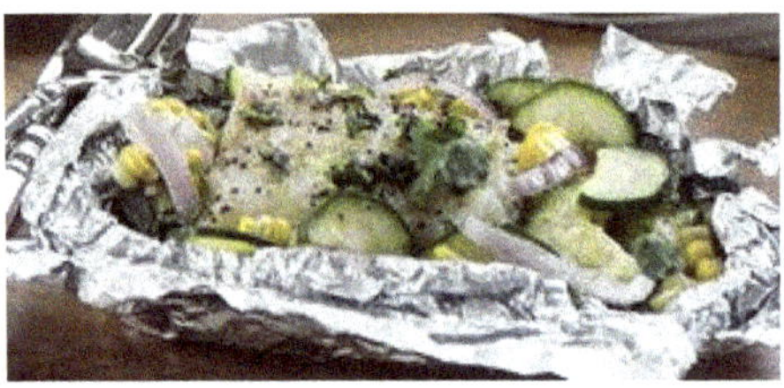

(Prepping time: 10 minutes | Cooking time: 15 minutes | For 2 servings)

Ingredients

- 24-ounces cod fillets, skin removed

- 1 tablespoon of blackening spices
- 2 zucchinis, sliced lengthwise from to form ribbon
- ½ a tablespoon of olive oil

How To

1. Season the fish fillets with blackening spice
2. Wrap each fish fillets with zucchini ribbons
3. Place fish on a plate
4. Take a skillet and place it over medium heat
5. Pour oil and allow the oil to heat up
6. Add wrapped fish to the skillet and cook each side for 4 minutes
7. Serve and enjoy!

Nutritional Values (Per Serving)

- Calories: 329
- Fat: 23g
- Carbohydrates: 2g
- Protein: 41g
- Saturated Fat: 6g
- Sodium: 978mg
- Fiber: 0.4g

Warm Vegetable And Coconut Meal

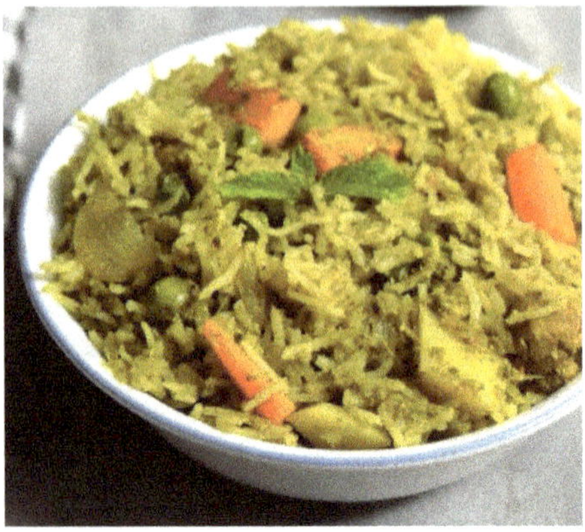

(Prepping time: 10 minutes | Cooking time: 25 minutes | For 4 servings)

Ingredients

- 1 tablespoon sunflower oil
- 1 medium brown onion, finely chopped
- 1 clove fresh garlic, crushed
- 1 teaspoon fresh ginger, finely grated
- 1 fresh red chili, thinly sliced
- ½ teaspoon ground coriander
- 1/8 teaspoon dried saffron
- 1 cup of low-fat coconut milk
- 2 teaspoon of fish sauce
- 1 medium lemon, cut into wedges
- 17 ounce of raw pumpkin, butternut, cut up into 1-inch pieces
- 14 ounce of potatoes, cut up into 1-inch pieces
- 7 ounce of green beans, cut up into thirds
- 1 medium red capsicum, cut into 1-inch pieces
- ½ a cup of fresh coriander, chopped

How To

1. Place a large saucepan over medium-high heat
2. Add oil and allow the oil to heat up.
3. Add onion and keep stirring them for 5 minutes.
4. Add ginger, garlic, ground coriander, chili, and saffron.
5. Cook for 1 minute until a nice fragrance develops.
6. Add coconut milk, 1 cup of water, and fish sauce to the mix.
7. Bring it to a boil.
8. Once boiling point is reached, add Potato and pumpkin.
9. Lower the heat and bring it to a simmer.
10. Simmer for 8-10 minutes
11. Add beans and capsicum. Cover and simmer for 5 minutes more.
12. Stir in half of the fresh coriander, sprinkling the remaining coriander on
13. top.
14. Serve with a lemon wedge.
15. Enjoy!

Nutritional Values (Per Serving)

- Calories: 235
- Fat: 17g
- Carbohydrates: 19g
- Protein: 5g
- Saturated Fat: 5g
- Sodium: 250 mg
- Fiber: 6g

Protein-Packed Bean Balls

(Prepping time: 10 minutes | Cooking time: 0 minutes | For 4 servings)

Ingredients

- ½ cup of dates
- ½ cup dried berries and cherries
- ½ cup ground almonds
- 2 tablespoons cocoa
- 3 ¾ cups of black beans
- Zest of 1 small orange
- As for topping
- Cocoa
- Coconut
- Toasted Pistachios

How To

1. Take a food processor and add dates, ground almond, cherries, cocoa, black beans, and orange zest.
2. Process until chopped.
3. Using your hands, make balls out of the mixture.
4. Garnish the balls with toasted cocoa, pistachios, and coconut.
5. Serve and enjoy!

Nutritional Values (Per Serving)

- Calories: 366
- Fat: 14g
- Carbohydrates: 96g
- Protein: 8g

- Saturated Fat: 3g
- Sodium: 228 mg
- Fiber: 10g

Wholesome Potato And Vegan Sauce

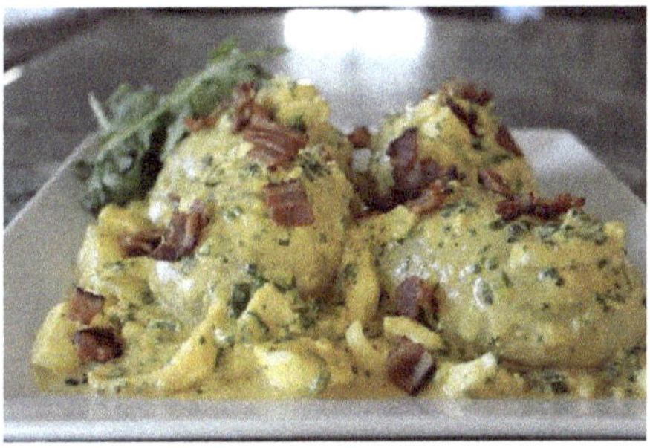

(Prepping time: 10 minutes | Cooking time: 30 minutes | For 4 servings)

Ingredients

- 2 pounds baby potatoes, halved
- 3 tablespoons canola oil
- 1 cup cashews, raw and soaked in warm water overnight
- 3 tablespoons lemon juice
- ½ teaspoon chili powder
- ½ teaspoon sweet paprika
- ½ teaspoon powdered garlic
- 1 teaspoon sea salt, regular or coarse, divided
- ¼ teaspoon pepper
- ¼ cup nutritional yeast
- ½ jalapeno chili, chopped and seeded

How To

1. Preheat your Oven to 450 degrees Fahrenheit.
2. In a bowl, mix together ½ teaspoon of salt, ¼ teaspoon of pepper, and
3. oil.
4. Take a rimmed baking sheet and spread potatoes evenly.
5. Spread the seasoning mix over the potatoes
6. Roast for 30 minutes.
7. In a blender, add lemon juice, chili powder, paprika, cashews, cumin,
8. garlic powder, yeast, jalapeno, and remaining sea salt.
9. Add 1 cup of water.
10. Mix well to puree.
11. Transfer the mix to a 2-quart saucepan and simmer over low heat for 5 minutes.
12. Transfer the sauce to a bowl and serve with roasted potatoes.

Nutritional Values (Per Serving)

- Calories: 380
- Fat: 18g
- Carbohydrates: 47g
- Protein: 10g
- Saturated Fat: 3g
- Sodium: 120 mg
- Fiber: 2g

Desserts

Cherry Tart

(Prepping Time: 30 minutes | Cooking Time: 8 minutes | For 16 servings)

Ingredients

- 9" pie crust
- 6 cup(s)s cherries, stemmed and pitted
- 2 tablespoon(s) + 2 teaspoon(s) powdered Stevia
- 3 tablespoon(s) cornstarch
- 1/2 cup(s)s water
- 3 oz low fat cream cheese, softened

How To

1. Bake the pie crust and set aside to cool.
2. Mash enough cherries to fill one cup(s).
3. In a saucepan over medium heat, add the cherries, the powdered Stevia, the cornstarch, and the water. Stir well to mix.
4. Stir often until the mixture comes to a boil and thickens. Cook for a minute after that.
5. Remove from heat and set aside to cool.
6. Put the cream cheese in a bowl and beat with a hand mixer until smooth.
7. Spread on the crust, making sure to cover the sides and the bottom.
8. Arrange the rest of the cherries on top of the cream cheese.
9. Pour the cooked mixture over the cherries and smooth.

10. Cover with Saran wrap and chill for a minimum of 3 hours before serving.

Nutritional Values (Per Serving)

- Calories: 103
- Fat: 4g
- Saturated Fat: 1.33g
- Trans Fat: 0g
- Carbohydrates: 16g
- Fiber: 1.5g
- Sodium: 93mg
- Protein: 1.5g

Peanut Butter Blizzard

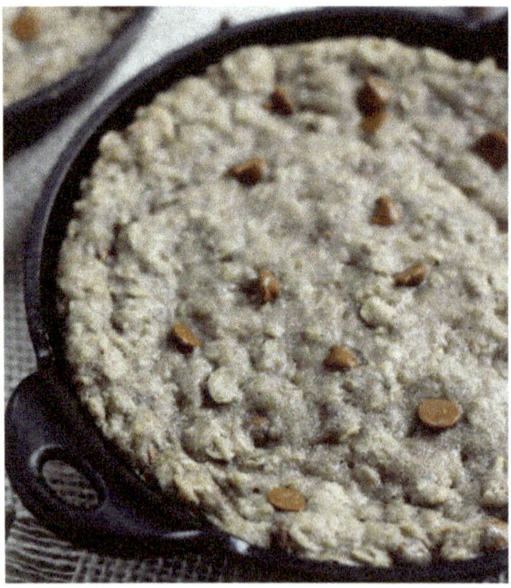

(Prepping Time: 5 mins. +overnight freezing. | Cooking Time: 5 minutes | For 12 servings)

Ingredients

- 6 bananas
- 1 tablespoon(s) almond milk
- 4 tablespoon(s) low fat peanut butter

How To

1. Peel the bananas and thickly slice them.
2. Freeze overnight.
3. Put the bananas and the milk in a high-speed blender. Let sit for 5 minutes.
4. Blend until they form a cream.
5. Add the peanut butter and blend again until the mix resembles soft serve.
6. Serve on its own or on fruit.

Nutritional Values (Per Serving)

- Calories: 85
- Fat: 2.3g
- Saturated Fat: 0.4g
- Trans Fat: 0g
- Carbohydrates: 16g
- Fiber: 2g
- Sodium: 34mg
- Protein: 2g

Strawberry Lemon Donuts

(Prepping Time: 15 minutes | Cooking Time: 10 minutes | For 10 servings)

Ingredients

- 1 cup(s) whole wheat flour
- 1/3 cup(s) Powdered Stevia
- 3/4 teaspoon(s) baking powder
- 3/4 teaspoon(s) baking soda
- 1/4 teaspoon(s) salt
- 1 egg
- 1/2 cup(s) low-fat yogurt
- 1 tablespoon(s) canola oil
- zest of one lemon
- 1 tablespoon(s) lemon juice
- 1 1/2 cup(s) fresh strawberries

How To

1. Preheat your oven to 375F.
2. Spray a doughnut pan with cooking spray.
3. Mix all of the dry ingredients in a bowl.
4. In another bowl mix all the wet ingredients apart from the fruit.
5. Mix the dry mix with the wet until you get a smooth batter
6. Fold in the fruit gently.
7. Drop 2 tablespoon(s) of the batter in each mold
8. Bake for 10 minutes, until your donuts are golden brown.

Nutritional Values (Per Serving)

- Calories: 82

- Fat: 2.8g
- Saturated Fat: 0.6g
- Trans Fat: 0g
- Carbohydrates: 13g
- Fiber: 3g
- Sodium: 170 mg
- Protein: 3g

Sweet Yogurt Dip

(Prepping Time: 5 minutes | Cooking Time: 5 minutes | For 32 servings)

Ingredients

- 1 cup(s) vanilla low-fat yogurt
- 3 tablespoon(s) sugar free maple syrup
- 1 cup(s) light cool whip

How To

1. Mix all of the ingredients together thoroughly.
2. Serve along with fruit, desserts, or breadsticks.
3. Store in an airtight container in the fridge.

Nutritional Values (Per Serving)

- Calories: 12
- Fat: 0.4g
- Saturated Fat: 0.3g
- Trans Fat: 0g

- Carbohydrates: 2g
- Fiber: 0g
- Sodium: 12g
- Protein: 0g

Chocolate Pancakes

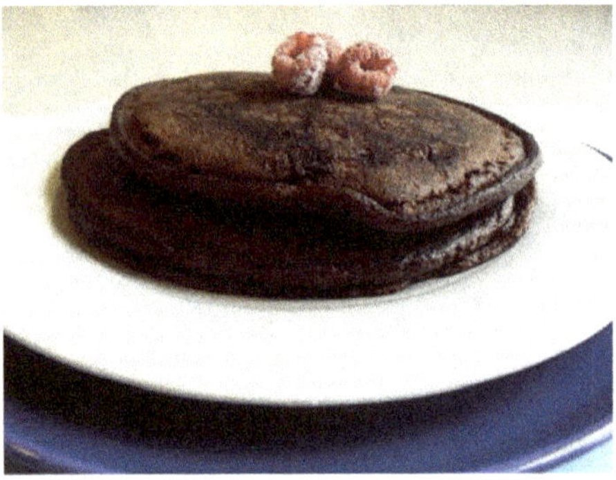

(Prepping Time: 15 minutes | Cooking Time: 30 minutes | For 16 servings)

Ingredients

- 2 1/2 cup(s)s whole wheat Flour
- 2 teaspoon(s) baking soda
- 4 tablespoon(s) Splenda
- 2 cup(s)s 2% milk
- 1 egg white
- 2 tablespoon(s) Vanilla extract
- 4 tablespoon(s) unsweetened cocoa

How To

1. Mix the dry ingredients in a bowl.
2. In another bowl, beat the milk, egg white, and the vanilla until even.
3. Mix into the dry ingredients and beat until you make a smooth batter
4. Heat a non-stick pan over high heat and spray with cooking spray.
5. Take a ladleful of the mix for each pancake and pour on the skillet.
6. Cook until bubbles start to form on the top side.
7. Flip with a spatula and cook for a minute on the other side.
8. Serve hot with toppings of your liking (calories and points not included)

Nutritional Values (Per Serving)

- Calories: 89
- Fat: 1.3g
- Saturated Fat: 0.6g
- Trans Fat: 0g
- Carbohydrates: 16g
- Fiber: 2g
- Sodium: 176mg
- Protein: 4g

Lime Muffins

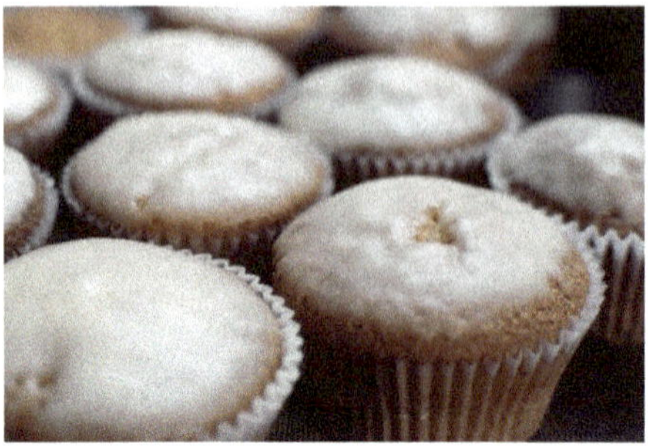

(Prepping Time: 20 minutes | Cooking Time: 15 minutes (per batch) | For 32 muffins)

Ingredients

- *For the Muffins:*
- 6 oz 20% margarine
- 5 oz powdered Stevia
- 4 Eggs
- 3 cup(s)s whole-wheat flour
- 1 cup(s) almond milk
- Zest of 4 limes
- 1/2 teaspoon(s) salt
- 3 teaspoon(s) baking powder
- *For the glaze:* (1 teaspoon(s) of per muffin)
- 1/2 cup(s) fresh lime juice
- 6 tablespoon(s) icing sugar

How To

1. For the muffins:

2. Preheat your oven at 400F

3. Line a muffin tray with muffin paper

4. In a mixing bowl, add the margarine, the Stevia, and the eggs and mix well until evenly combined.

5. Mix in the flour, the milk, the zest, salt, and the baking powder. Use a hand mixer to beat until it's a smooth batter.

6. Divide among the muffin cup(s)s, filling each wrapper about halfway through.

7. Bake for 15 minutes per batch.

8. *For the glaze:*

9. Whisk the lime juice and the icing sugar well.

10. When you get the muffins out of the oven, use a fork to prick the tops and drop one teaspoon(s) of the glaze on top of each muffin.

11. Allow to fully cool before serving.

Nutritional Values (Per Serving)

- Calories: 100
- Fat: 5.2g
- Saturated Fat: 3g
- Trans Fat: 0.1g
- Carbohydrates: 15.6g
- Fiber: 0.4g
- Sodium: 78mg
- Protein: 2.2g

Strawberry Tart

(Prepping Time: 30 minutes | Cooking Time: 8 minutes | For 8 servings)

Ingredients

- 9" pie crust
- 6 cups strawberries
- 2 tablespoons+ 2 teaspoons stevia
- 3 tablespoons cornstarch
- 1/2 cups water
- 3 oz low-fat cream cheese, softened

How to

1. Bake the pie crust and allow to cool.
2. Mash enough strawberries to fill one cup.
3. In a saucepan over medium heat, add the berries, the stevia, the cornstarch, and the water. Stir well to mix.
4. Keep stirring until it comes to a boil and the mixture thickens. After it boils, cook for a minute.
5. Remove from heat and allow to cool.
6. In a bowl, add the cream cheese and beat with a hand mixer until smooth.
7. Spread on the sides and bottom of the crust.
8. Slice the rest of the strawberries and arrange on top of the cream cheese.
9. Pour the cooked mixture over the strawberries and smooth.

9.6.1 Cover with shrink wrap and chill for a minimum of 3 hours before serving.

Nutritional Values (Per Serving)

- Calories: 149
- Fat: 6.4g
- Saturated Fat: 1g
- Trans Fat: 0.1g
- Carbohydrates: 20.6g
- Fiber: 2.4g
- Sodium: 176mg
- Protein: 3.1g

Rhubarb Granita

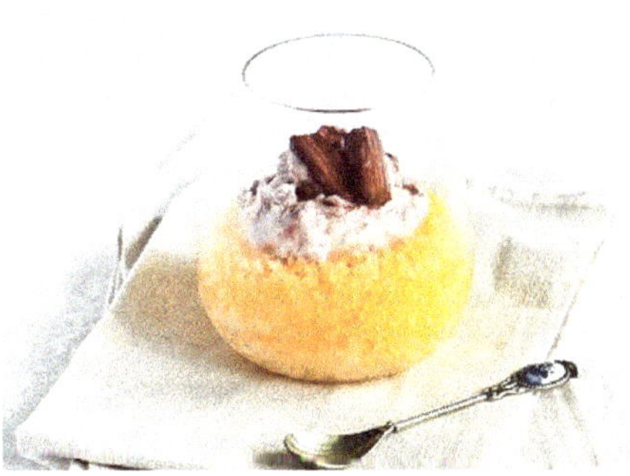

(Prepping Time: 25 min | Cooking Time: 10 min | For 6 servings)

Ingredients

- ½ cup unsweetened applesauce
- 4 cups sliced rhubarb
- 3 cups water
- 1 tablespoon fresh mint leaves

- 1 cup blueberries
- ½ cup raspberries

How to

1. Add rhubarb, water, unsweetened applesauce, mint leaves, and blueberries in a pan.
2. Cook for about 10 minutes and stir occasionally.
3. Take out and strain the mixture in a dish.
4. Place the dish in freezer for half an hour.
5. Take out and scrap the mixture.
6. Again put it in freezer for 1 hour.
7. Take out and top it with raspberries.
8. Serve and enjoy!

Nutritional Values (Per Serving)

- Calories: 45
- Fat: 0.3g
- Saturated Fat: 0g
- Trans Fat: 0.1g
- Carbohydrates: 10.8g
- Fiber: 3g
- Sodium: 8mg
- Protein: 1.1g

Apple Crisp

(Prepping Time: 10 minutes | Cooking Time: 45 minutes | For 16 servings)

Ingredients

- 7 medium apples, cored& peeled, thinly sliced
- 1 tablespoon whole-wheat flour
- 1 teaspoon cinnamon
- A pinch of salt
- 1/4 cup water
- 9oz cake mix
- 3/4 cup quick oats
- 1/3 cup margarine 20% fat, softened
- 1 1/4 cup brown sugar Splenda
- 1/4 teaspoon baking powder
- 1/4 teaspoon baking soda

How to

1. Layer the apple slices on the bottom of a shallow baking dish.
2. Combine the 1 cup of brown sugar, flour, salt, and cinnamon in a bowl and mix until evenly combined, then sprinkle over the apples.
3. Drizzles over the mixture with water.
4. In a mixer bowl, add the cake mix, butter, oats, remaining sugar, baking soda, and baking powder until well combined.
5. Pour the mixture over the apples.
6. Bake for around 45 minutes until the top is golden brown.
7. Serve warm.

Nutritional Values (Per Tablespoon)

- Calories: 137
- Fat: 4.2g
- Saturated Fat: 0.9g
- Trans Fat: 0.1g

- Carbohydrates: 29.2g
- Fiber: 5g
- Sodium: 122mg
- Protein: 1.4g

Banana Cookie Blizzard

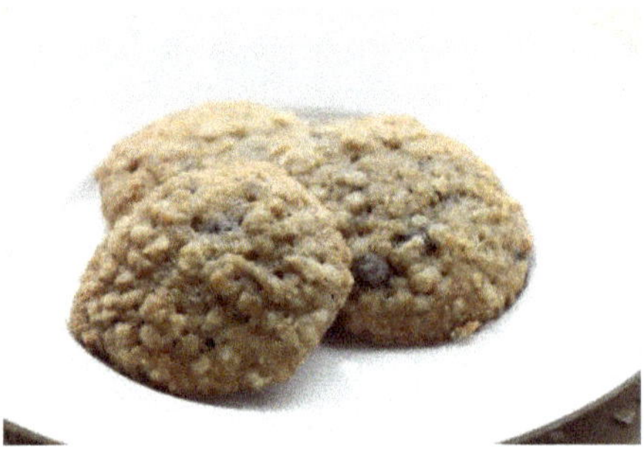

(Prepping Time: 5 mins. +overnight freezing. | Cooking Time: 5 minutes | For 4 servings)

Ingredients

- 6 bananas
- 1 tablespoon almond milk
- 4 tablespoons cookie dough

How to

1. Peel the bananas and cut them up into small chunks.
2. Freeze overnight.
3. Put the bananas and the milk in a food processor and blend until they form a cream.

4. Add the cookie dough and blend again until the mix resembles soft serve.
5. Eat on each own or over cookie dough balls.

Nutritional Values (Per Serving)

- Calories: 191.5
- Fat: 2.7g
- Saturated Fat: 1.2g
- Trans Fat: 0.1g
- Carbohydrates: 43.2g
- Fiber: 4.8g
- Sodium: 38mg
- Protein: 2.4g

Rainbow Kabobs

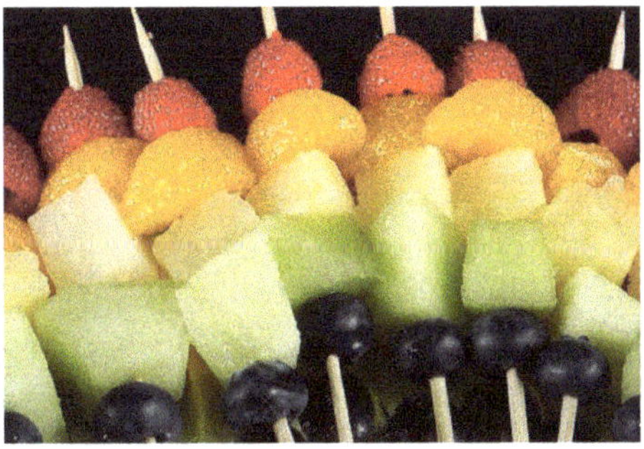

(Prepping Time: 15 minutes | Cooking Time: 5 minutes | For 12 Servings)

Ingredients

- 6 strawberries, sliced in half or 12 raspberries

- 12 mango cubes
- 6 orange slices, cut in half
- 12 pineapple chunks or 12 banana slices
- 12 kiwi slices
- 12 blueberries
- 3 plums, cut in fourths

How To

1. Wash the fruit and cut them into the shape needed,
2. Thread the fruit pieces on skewers in the order of the colors of the rainbow.
3. Serve immediately along with yogurt dip if you like (points and calories not included)

Nutritional Values (Per Serving)

- Calories: 85
- Fat: 0.5g
- Saturated Fat: 0g
- Trans Fat: 0g
- Carbohydrates: 21.5g
- Fiber: 3.5g
- Sodium: 2mg
- Protein: 1.3g

Yogurt-covered fruit

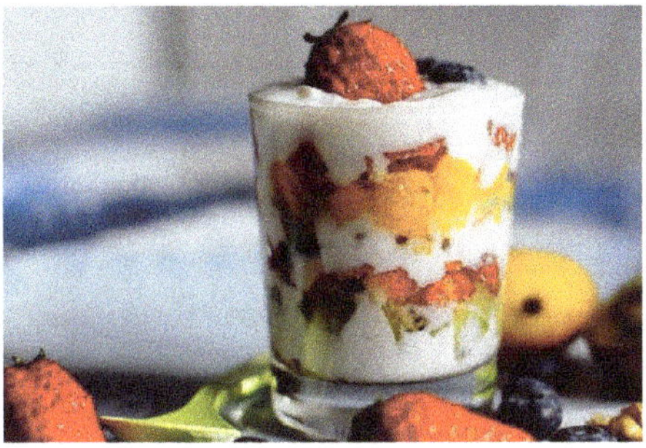

(Prepping Time: 30 minutes | Cooking Time: 60 minutes | For 12 Servings)

Ingredients

- 12 strawberries
- 1 mango, peeled, pitted, and cut in chunks
- 2 peaches, peeled, pitted, and cut in chunks
- 3 kiwis, peeled and sliced
- 2 cup(s)s fat free Greek yogurt
- 1 teaspoon(s) vanilla extract

How To

1. Mix the vanilla extract with the yogurt in a bowl.
2. Line a baking sheet that fits in your freezer with parchment.
3. Dip the fruit in the yogurt and arrange on the sheet.
4. Freeze for 3 hours before serving.

Nutritional Values (Per Serving)

- Calories: 51
- Fat: 0.3g
- Saturated Fat: .1g
- Trans Fat: 0g
- Carbohydrates: 10g

- Fiber: 1g
- Sodium: 9mg
- Protein: 3g

Banana Mousse

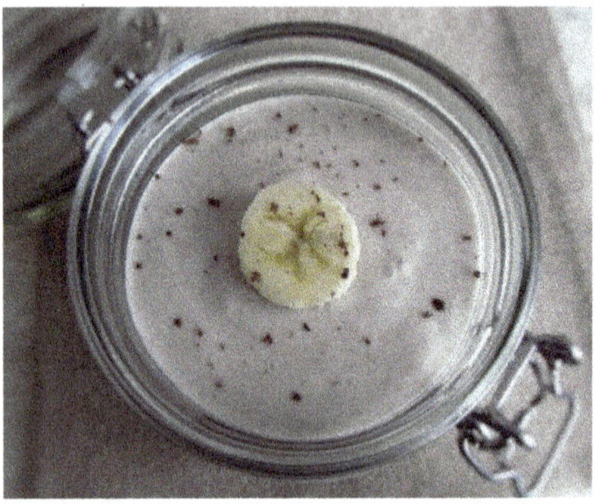

(Prepping Time: 5 minutes | Cooking Time: 5 minutes | For 24 Servings)

Ingredients

- 2 Boxes Sugar Free& Fat Free Instant Banana Pudding Mix
- 6 Cup(s)s 2% Milk
- 16 oz Fat Free Cool Whip

How To

1. Using a mixer, whisk the pudding with the milk until it starts to thicken.
2. Add the cool whip and whisk until it's smooth.
3. Divide into 24 cup(s)s.
4. Refrigerate for at least two hours before serving.

Nutritional Values (Per Serving)

- Calories: 54
- Fat: 1.2g
- Saturated Fat: 0.7g
- Trans Fat: 0.1g
- Carbohydrates: 8.2g
- Fiber: 0.2g
- Sodium: 184mg
- Protein: 2.3g

Cookie Dough Pancakes

(Prepping Time: 15 minutes | Cooking Time: 30 minutes | For 12 Servings)

Ingredients

- 2 cup(s)s whole wheat flour
- 2 cup(s)s oats
- 4 1/2 teaspoon(s) vanilla extract
- 1 tablespoon(s) powdered Stevia
- 3/4 teaspoon(s) salt
- 2 tablespoon(s) baking powder
- ½ teaspoon(s) baking soda
- 3 cup(s) low fat milk
- 6 tablespoon(s) unsweetened chocolate chips

How To

1. Mix the dry ingredients in a bowl.
2. In another bowl, beat the wet ingredients until combined.
3. Mix into the dry ingredients and beat until you make a smooth batter

4. Heat a non-stick pan over high heat and spray with cooking spray.
5. Take a ladleful of the mix for each pancake and pour on the skillet.
6. Cook until bubbles start to form on the top side.
7. Flip with a spatula and cook for a minute on the other side.
8. Serve hot.

Nutritional Values (Per Serving)

- Calories: 168
- Fat: 5.2g
- Saturated Fat: 2.3g
- Trans Fat: 0.1g
- Carbohydrates: 31g
- Fiber: 6g
- Sodium: 230mg
- Protein: 8g

Peach Tart

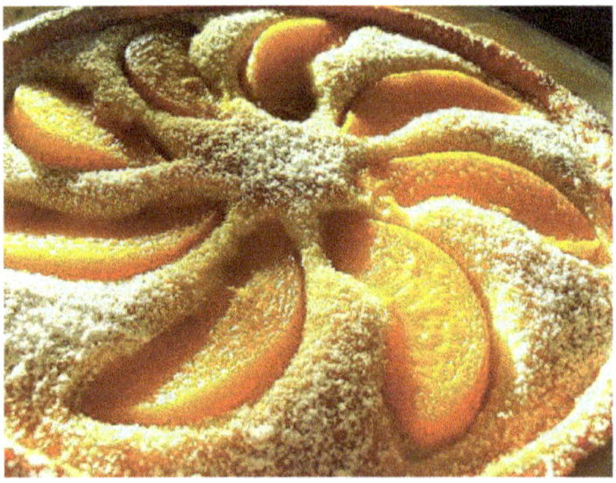

(Prepping Time: 30 minutes | Cooking Time: 8 minutes | For 16 Servings)

Ingredients

- 9" pie crust
- 6 cup(s)s peaches, peeled and pitted

- 2 tablespoon(s) + 2 teaspoon(s) powdered Stevia
- 3 tablespoon(s) cornstarch
- 1/2 cup(s)s water
- 3 oz low fat cream cheese, softened

How To

1. Bake the pie crust and set aside to cool.
2. Mash enough peaches to fill one cup(s).
3. In a saucepan over medium heat, add the peaches, the powdered Stevia, the cornstarch, and the water. Stir well to mix.
4. Stir often until the mixture comes to a boil and thickens. Cook for a minute after that.
5. Remove from heat and set aside to cool.
6. Put the cream cheese in a bowl and beat with a hand mixer until smooth.
7. Spread on the crust, making sure to cover the sides and the bottom.
8. Arrange the rest of the peaches on top of the cream cheese.
9. Pour the cooked mixture over the peaches and smooth.
10. Cover with Saran wrap and chill for a minimum of 3 hours before serving.

Nutritional Values (Per Serving)

- Calories: 103
- Fat: 4g
- Saturated Fat: 1.33g
- Trans Fat: 0g
- Carbohydrates: 16g
- Fiber: 1.5g
- Sodium: 93mg
- Protein: 1.5g

Cookie Dough Balls

(Prepping Time: 5 minutes | Cooking Time: 15 minutes | For 24 Servings)

Ingredients

- 24 unsalted cashews
- 2 tablespoons rolled oats
- 2 tablespoons whole wheat flour (other flours may work)
- A pinch of salt
- 2 teaspoons cane sugar
- 1/4 teaspoon vanilla extract
- 1 teaspoon maple syrup
- 2 tablespoon mini dark choc chips

How To

1. Place the oats and cashews in a food processor and blend until crumbly.
2. Add the sugar, salt, and flour and keep blending for a couple of seconds,
3. Add the maple syrup and the vanilla and blend until evenly combined. If it's too dry, add a teaspoon of water. The dough should be sticky.
4. Add the chips and blend by hand.
5. Form balls, each about half a teaspoon of dough
6. Store in the freezer.

Nutritional Values (Per Serving)

- Calories: 17
- Fat: 0.8g
- Saturated Fat: 0.2g
- Trans Fat: 0.1g

- Carbohydrates: 2.2g
- Fiber: 0.2g
- Sodium: 24mg
- Protein: 0.3g

Fruit& Nut Cookies

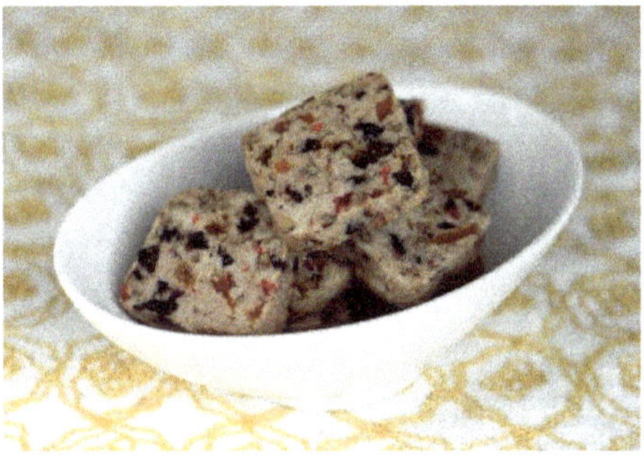

(Prepping Time: 5 minutes | Cooking Time: 15 minutes | For 30 Servings)

Ingredients

- 4 ripe bananas, mashed
- 4 tablespoons almond milk
- 4 tablespoons sugar-free apricot preserves
- 1/2 cup craisins
- 1/2 cup apricots, peeled and seeded
- 2 cups oatmeal
- 1 teaspoon salt
- 1 teaspoon vanilla
- 1 cup walnuts, chopped

How To

1. Preheat oven to 375F.

2. In a large bowl, mix all of the ingredients and blend until they're evenly mixed.
3. Using a tablespoon, drop one spoonful per cookie on a parchment-lined baking sheet.
4. Bake for 13 minutes until they're golden brown.

Nutritional Values (Per Cookie)

- Calories: 69
- Fat: 3.4g
- Saturated Fat: 0.6g
- Polyunsaturated Fat: 0.1 g
- Carbohydrates: 9g
- Fiber: 1.3g
- Sodium: 78mg
- Protein: 1.9g

Choco Sorbet

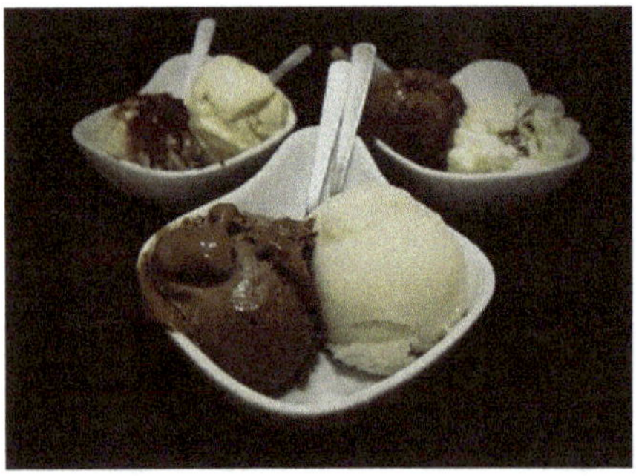

(Prepping Time: 25 min | Cooking Time: 5 min | For 12 Servings)

Ingredients

- 4 cups water
- 1 cup unsweetened cocoa powder

- 2 tablespoons olive oil
- 1 cup dark chocolate, chopped
- 1 cup swerve
- ½ cup chocolate syrup
- ½ cup chocolate chips

How To

1. Boil water, cocoa powder, dark chocolate, and swerve in a pan over medium-high heat. Beat continuously.
2. Lower the heat and let it simmer for about 30 seconds.
3. Transfer into heat-proof bowl and refrigerate for about 6 hours.
4. Then, put the mixture in an ice cream maker and add oil. Process it according to manufacturer's directions.
5. After that, refrigerate it again for about 2 hours and take out.
6. Add chocolate syrup and chocolate chips on the top and serve.

Nutritional Values (Per Serving)

- Calories: 155
- Fat: 8g
- Saturated Fat: 4g
- Trans Fat: 3.8g
- Carbohydrates: 21.9g
- Fiber: 3.2g
- Sodium: 29mg
- Protein: 2.8g

Chocolate Mousse

(Prepping Time: 5 minutes | Cooking Time: 5 minutes | For 12 Servings)

Ingredients

- 1 box sugar-free & fat-free instant chocolate pudding mix
- 3 cups 2% Milk
- 8oz fat-free cool whip

How To

1. Using a mixer, beat the pudding mix the milk until it starts to thicken.
2. Add the cool whip and beat until it's evenly incorporated.
3. Divide into 12 cups.
4. Chill for at least two hours before serving.

Nutritional Values (Per Serving)

- Calories: 54
- Fat: 1.2g
- Saturated Fat: 0.7g
- Trans Fat: 0.1g
- Carbohydrates: 8.2g
- Fiber: 0.2g
- Sodium: 184mg
- Protein: 2.3g

Raspberry Tart

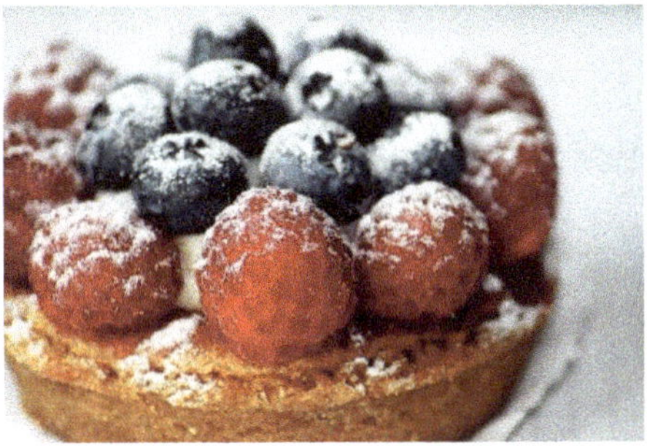

(Prepping Time: 30 minutes | Cooking Time: 8 minutes | For 16 servings)

Ingredients

- 9" pie crust
- 6 cup(s)s Raspberries
- 2 tablespoon(s) + 2 teaspoon(s) powdered Stevia
- 3 tablespoon(s) cornstarch
- 1/2 cup(s)s water
- 3 oz low fat cream cheese, softened

How To

1. Bake the pie crust and set aside to cool.
2. Mash enough Raspberries to fill one cup(s).
3. In a saucepan over medium heat, add the Raspberries, the powdered Stevia, the cornstarch, and the water. Stir well to mix.
4. Stir often until the mixture comes to a boil and thickens. Cook for a minute after that.
5. Remove from heat and set aside to cool.
6. Put the cream cheese in a bowl and beat with a hand mixer until smooth.

7. Spread on the crust, making sure to cover the sides and the bottom.
8. Arrange the rest of the Raspberries on top of the cream cheese.
9. Pour the cooked mixture over the Raspberries and smooth.
10. Cover with Saran wrap and chill for a minimum of 3 hours before serving.

Nutritional Values (Per Serving)

- Calories: 103
- Fat: 4g
- Saturated Fat: 1.33g
- Trans Fat: 0g
- Carbohydrates: 16g
- Fiber: 1.5g
- Sodium: 93mg
- Protein: 1.5g

Lemon Bars

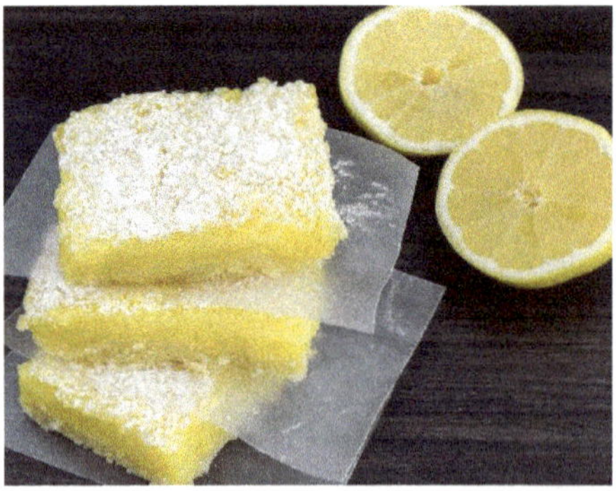

(Prepping Time: 15 minutes | Cooking Time: 30 minutes + an additional 4 hours to chill | For 12 servings)

Ingredients

- For the Crust:
- 3/4 cup(s) sugar-free graham cracker crumbs
- 2 tablespoon(s) 20% margarine
- For the Cream:
- 6 oz light cream cheese, softened
- 3/4 cup(s) plain nonfat Greek yogurt, at room temperature
- 2 large eggs, at room temperature
- 1 egg yolk, at room temperature
- 1/6 cup(s) Stevia
- 1/3 cup(s) lemon juice
- 1 tablespoon(s) lemon zest
- 1 teaspoon(s) vanilla extract

How To

1. Preheat your oven to 300F
2. Line an 8x8" baking pan with parchment paper, making sure the paper overhangs.
3. For the crust:
4. Mix the graham cracker crumbs with the margarine in a bowl until they are evenly combined.
5. Press the mixture on the bottom of the baking pan to form the crust.
6. Bake for 8 minutes.
7. Remove from the oven and set aside to cool.
8. For the cream:
9. In a mixing bowl, beat the cream cheese with a hand mixer on high for about 1 minute.
10. Add the yogurt and beat until combined.

11. Add the eggs and the egg yolk and beat until combined.
12. Mix in the sugar, the lemon juice, lemon zest, and the vanilla extract and beat until combined.
13. Pour over the crust and bake for 30 minutes. If the middle jiggles bake for another 2-5 minutes.
14. Allow to cool on a wire rack for a minimum of 30 minutes, then refrigerate for at least 4 hours.
15. Cut before serving.

Nutritional Values (Per Serving)

- Calories: 95
- Fat: 6.1g
- Saturated Fat: 3g
- Trans Fat: 0g
- Carbohydrates: 7g
- Fiber: 0g
- Sodium: 118mg
- Protein: 4g

Low Carb Banana Pancakes

(Prepping Time: 5 minutes | Cooking Time: 5 minutes | For 18 servings)

Ingredients

- 3 large bananas
- 6 eggs
- 1 1/2 teaspoon(s) vanilla extract
- 1 1/2 teaspoon(s) baking powder

- 3 teaspoon(s) cinnamon

How To

1. Mash the banana with a fork.
2. Whisk the eggs and add the banana, the baking powder, the cinnamon, and the vanilla. Whisk until you get a smooth batter.
3. In a non-stick pan over medium heat melt half a tablespoon(s) margarine.
4. Take a ladleful of the batter and pour in the pan.
5. Cook for 1 minute until the top of the pancake begins to bubble.
6. Flip the pancake and cook the other side for another minute.
7. Repeat until you finish with the batter.

Nutritional Values (Per Serving)

- Calories: 44
- Fat: 1.5g
- Saturated Fat: 0.5g
- Trans Fat: 0g
- Carbohydrates: 6g
- Fiber: 1g
- Sodium: 21mg
- Protein: 2g

Raisin Almond Cookies

(Prepping Time: 5 minutes | Cooking Time: 15 minutes | For 30 cookies)

Ingredients

- 4 bananas, mashed
- 4 tablespoon(s) almond Milk
- 4 tablespoon(s) sugar free grape preserves
- 1 cup(s) raisins
- 2 cup(s)s Oatmeal
- 1 teaspoon(s) salt
- 1 teaspoon(s) vanilla
- 1 cup(s) almonds, chopped

How To

1. Preheat your oven to 375F.
2. In a mixing bowl, mix all of the ingredients and beat with a hand mixer until they are evenly combined.
3. Using a tablespoon(s) form a ball of dough, (1 spoonful per cookie) on a parchment-lined baking sheet.
4. Bake for 13 minutes until golden.

Nutritional Values (Per Serving)

- Calories: 31
- Fat: 0.6g
- Saturated Fat: 0.1g
- Trans Fat: 0g
- Carbohydrates: 8g
- Fiber: 1g
- Sodium: 80mg
- Protein: 1g

Chocolate Cake

(Prepping Time: 10 minutes | Cooking Time: 35 minutes | For 8 servings)

Ingredients

- 2/3 cup(s) stevia
- 1 cup(s) +2 tablespoon(s) all-purpose flour
- 2 tablespoon(s) cocoa powder
- 1 teaspoon(s) baking powder
- 1 teaspoon(s) baking soda
- 3 small egg whites
- 2/3 cup(s) skimmed milk
- 1/3 cup(s) unsweetened applesauce
- 1 1/3 teaspoon(s) vanilla extract
- 2/3 cup(s) boiling water

How To

1. Preheat your oven at 350F
2. Mix all of the dry ingredients in a mixing bowl.
3. Add the wet ingredients to the dry and mix with a whisk lightly until combined. The batter should be liquid.
4. Spray a springform pan with non-stick spray and pour in the batter.
5. Bake for 35 minutes.
6. Allow to completely cool before cutting.
7. Enjoy!

Nutritional Values (Per Serving)

- Calories: 107
- Fat: 2.4g

- Saturated Fat: 1g
- Trans Fat: 0g
- Carbohydrates: 19g
- Fiber: 1g
- Sodium: 188mg
- Protein: 5g

No-Flour Cookiesc

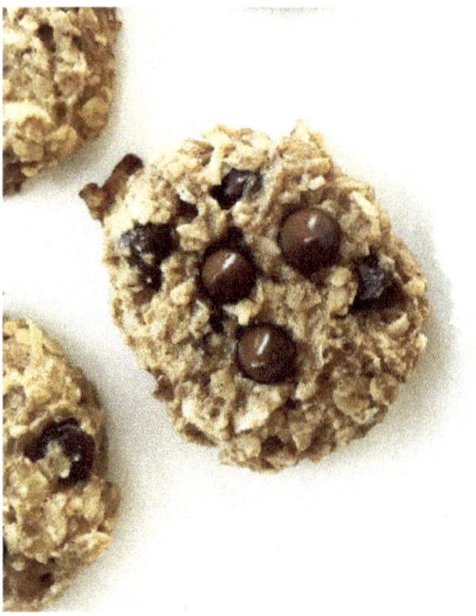

(Prepping Time: 10 minutes | Cooking Time: 15 minutes | For 24 cookies)

Ingredients

- 1 cup honey
- 2 eggs
- 1 cup peanut butter

How to

1. Preheat oven to 300F.
2. Mix ingredients with a mixer until you have a smooth dough
3. Line a baking sheet with parchment paper and roll a tablespoon of the dough in a ball for each cookie. Flatten each ball.
4. Bake for 15 minutes per batch until golden.

Nutritional Values (per cookie)

- Calories: 111
- Fat: 5.8g
- Saturated Fat: 1.3g
- Trans Fat: 0.1g
- Carbohydrates: 13.8g
- Fiber: 0.7g
- Sodium: 55mg
- Protein: 3.2g

No-Bake Cheesecake

(Prepping Time: 10 minutes | Cooking Time: 5 minutes+ chilling overnight. | For 8 servings)

Ingredients

- 1 9" Graham Crackers crust
- 4oz. fat-free cream cheese
- 1/2 cup cold hazelnut milk

- 1 tablespoon lemon juice
- 1/2 small box sugar-free instant vanilla pudding
- 4 oz. fat-free Cool Whip
- 1/2 can pie filling (Lite with the flavor of your choosing)

How to

1. Using a mixer, beat the cream cheese, milk, and lemon juice until smooth.
2. Add the pudding mix and mix until incorporated.
3. Fold in the cool whip.
4. Pour the cheese mixture into the pie crust and smooth over with a spatula.
5. Top with the pie filling.
6. Chill overnight before serving.

Nutritional Values (Per Serving)

- Calories: 112
- Fat: 6.1g
- Saturated Fat: 3.4g
- Trans Fat: 0.1g
- Carbohydrates: 11.4g
- Fiber: 0.4g
- Sodium: 78mg
- Protein: 1.7

Ricotta Mousse

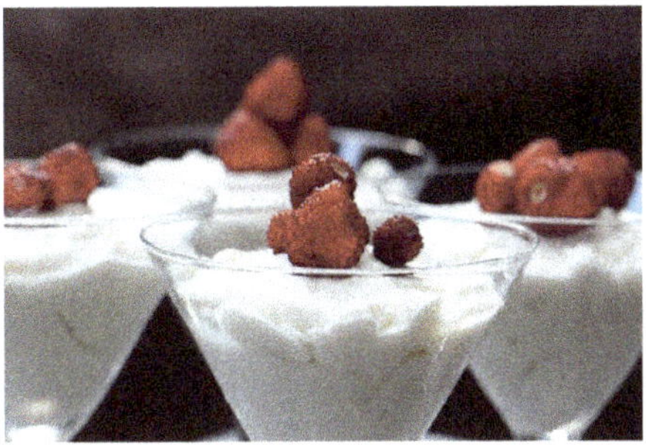

(Prepping Time: 10 min. | Cooking Time: 0 min | For 2 servings)

Ingredients

- 2 ½ cups of water, divided
- ½ teaspoon pure vanilla extract
- 1 cup ricotta cheese
- 2 teaspoons cocoa powder
- 2 teaspoons stevia powder
- ¼ cup blueberries

How to

1. Add ricotta cheese, cocoa powder, stevia powder, vanilla extract, and water in a bowl. Mix well.
2. Transfer the mixture into serving glasses and top with blueberries.
3. Refrigerate for about 6 hours and take out.
4. Serve with a smile and enjoy!

Nutritional Values (Per Serving)

- Calories: 189

- Fat: 10.1g
- Saturated Fat: 6.3g
- Trans Fat: 4.1g
- Carbohydrates: 10.1g
- Fiber: 1g
- Sodium: 164mg
- Protein: 14.6g

CPSIA information can be obtained
at www.ICGtesting.com
Printed in the USA
LVHW080808030122
707668LV00010B/273

9 781914 107931